WEIGHT SUCCESS

In Essence, You Make Weight Success Happen Like This ...

1 – *READ this Book (or at least read pages 12–68).* ✱

2 – *DO the Weight Success Method each day (typically takes less than eight minutes).*

3 – *THEN you'll be on the road to realizing lifelong Weight Success — that is, on the road to living most or all of your days in your desired healthy-weight range <u>and</u> deriving benefits, enjoyment, and fulfillment from it.*

✱ NOTE: You don't need to read this entire book to get started on your weight success journey. All you need to do is read pages 12–68 (which contains the Introduction and Chapters 1 and 2). Also, if you're one who dislikes extensive reading or dislikes reading more than a few paragraphs in a session, here's a suggestion. Commit to reading *one page each day.* By doing this you'll have pages 12–68 read in 60 days. A page can be read in about six minutes or less. So, an investment of six minutes reading time for each of sixty days would get the job done.

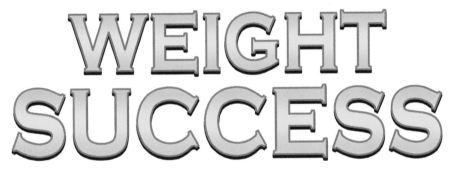

WEIGHT SUCCESS

A Guide to Living Your Life in Your Desired Weight Range
and Deriving Benefits and Enjoyment from It

John Correll

Fulfillment Press

U.S.A.

WEIGHT SUCCESS: A Guide to Living Your Life in Your Desired Weight Range and Deriving Benefits and Enjoyment from It

Fulfillment Press | U.S.A.

Printed in United States of America
ISBN: 978-1-938001-76-5
Amazon URL: amazon.com/dp/1938001761
Library of Congress Control Number: 2021904546
Version: TXT 2021-03 (6) | COV 2021-03 (3)
Cover, photographs, text creation, formatting, editing and proof reading by John Correll

Fulfillment Press specializes in the creation and publication of educational media for career and life fulfillment. The name *Fulfillment Press* is a publishing imprint and registered DBA, or assumed name, of Correll Consulting, LLC. The name *Weight Success Method™* is a trademarked name used by Correll Consulting, LLC to denote the weight management method described in this book. *World Weight Success Empowerment Series™* is also a trademarked name and is used by Correll Consulting, LLC to denote a book/E-book series.

John Correll enjoys walking, biking with his grandson, sight-seeing, creating photographs, book publishing, and reading American history and positive psychology. More on him can be found at:
correllconcepts.com/correll_bio.htm
(Note: This is not the same John Correll who creates the excellent kids' books.)

Dedicated to the Readers of this book. ~ May you live out your life in your desired weight range and strive to become the finest person you're capable of being and help others to do the same … and derive peace, joy, and fulfillment as a result.

Special thanks to my wife and life partner Janet for triggering my initial search for the cause of why a few people are succeeding at creating healthy-weight living while most are not.

Disclaimer: Before beginning any diet or weight management program, or making a major change to a present dietary program, a licensed physician should be consulted. If any information in this book should contradict or conflict with any prescription or advice of your physician or chosen dietary program, we recommend you ignore and do not apply whatever that conflicting information contained in this book might be. This book is not a dietary guide. It does not recommend a particular dietary program. It aims at a general audience. The Weight Success Method and other methods, suggestions, and statements contained in this book derive from the author's personal experiences, perspectives, and conclusions. They do not derive from scientific testing; therefore, it should not be assumed that these methods, suggestions, and statements will work for every person and in every situation. The author and publisher shall have neither liability nor responsibility to any person or entity with respect to any loss or damage caused, or alleged to have been caused, directly or indirectly, by the information contained in this book.

For additional resources and books by John Correll, go to: correllconcepts.com

Consulting Service – If your company or organization would like a keynote speaker or would like assistance in implementing the principles of the Weight Success Method in a customized program for clients or staff, go to: correllconcepts.com/consulting.pdf

SUCCESS is:

The act of creating a desired life-enhancing situation <u>and</u> deriving benefits, enjoyment, and fulfillment from it.

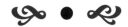

WEIGHT SUCCESS is:

Living most or all of one's days in one's desired healthy-weight range <u>and</u> deriving benefits, enjoyment, and fulfillment from it.

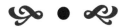

This book is about <u>creating</u> **WEIGHT SUCCESS**. To succeed at creating weight success you must apply a weight success program <u>and</u> you must do the program <u>every day</u>. The Weight Success Method presented in this book is such a program.

Table of Contents

If you're one who desires to succeed at putting your life on the track of lifelong healthy-weight living, and do it more easily and enjoyably than you've likely ever thought possible, this book is for **YOU.**

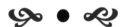

This book presents numerous new concepts. Some of these concepts are central to succeeding at healthy-weight living. These key concepts are restated throughout the book.
This restatement is **INTENTIONAL.**

SPECIAL EXTRA SECTION:
Why Most Persons Aren't Pursuing Weight Management

WEIGHT MANAGEMENT is <u>not</u> hard to do IF it's pursued the right way. So, why do most persons refuse to seriously pursue weight management? It's because they hold an *erroneous conception* of it. They view it ...

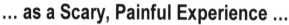

... as a Scary, Painful Experience ...

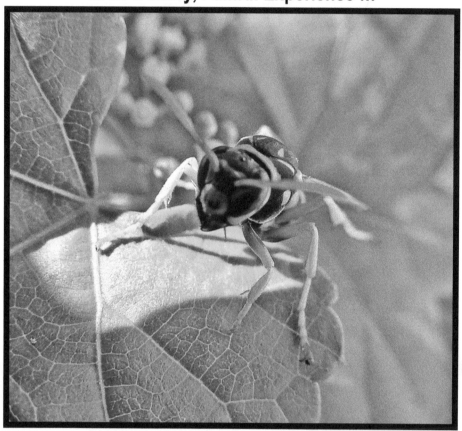

... or as an Endless Series of Problems and Dilemmas ...

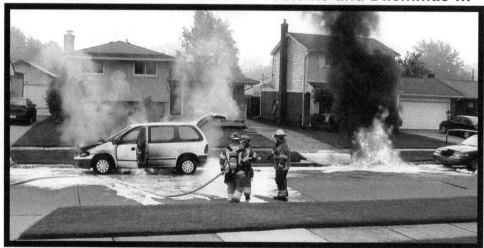

... or as a Daily Distasteful Activity ...

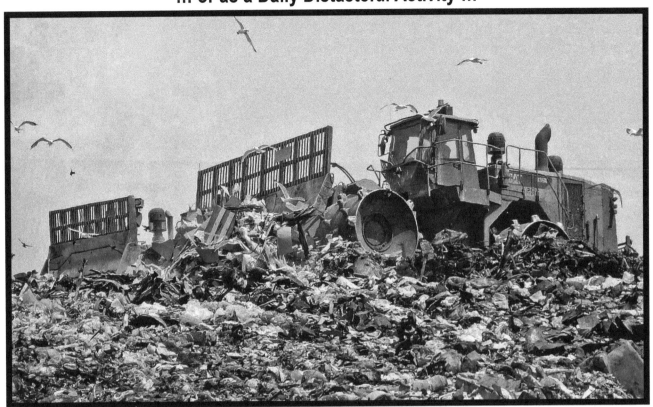

... or as a Sinking Journey to No-where Land ...

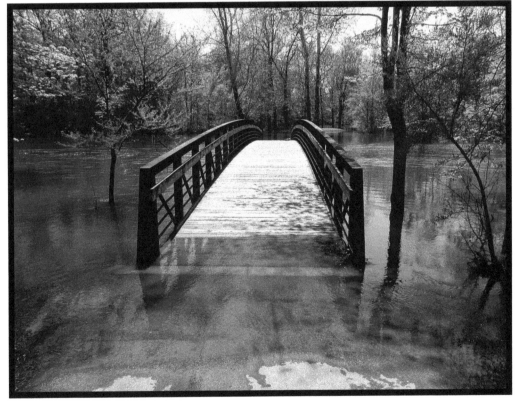

... or as Endless Eating like a Bird ...

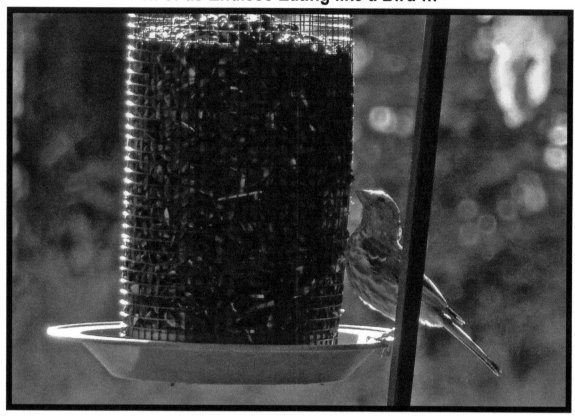

... or as Hours of Rigorous Daily Exercise.

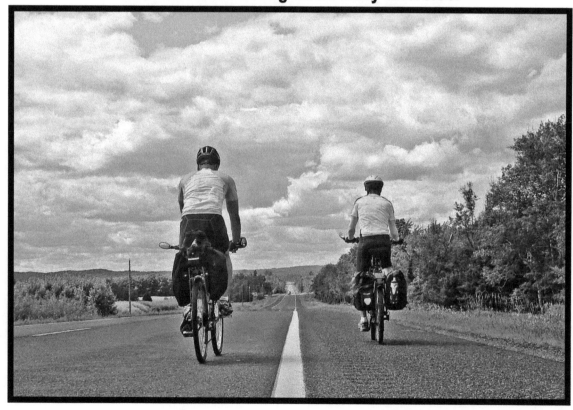

But, in actuality, it's <u>none</u> of those things!

To create maximal success in weight management, one must approach weight management with a certain *productive* outlook. Starting with Day 1, here's the outlook that will yield optimal results in your weight success pursuit.

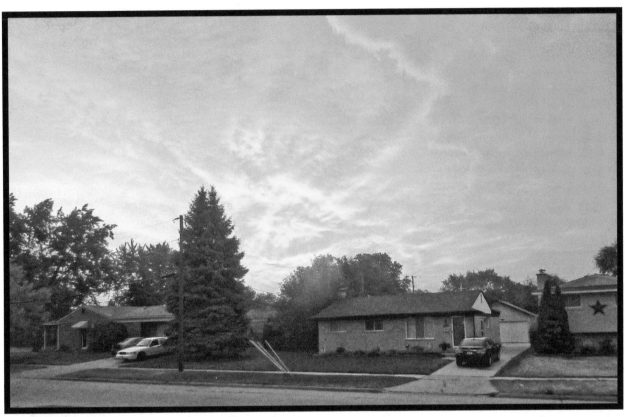

Today is the dawning of another great day in my **Weight Success Journey** *— a journey that includes healthy-weight living, daily victory, positive learning experiences, self-discovery epiphanies, numerous personal benefits,* <u>*and*</u> *daily eating enjoyment.*

With that outlook in mind, turn to the next page — and begin what will likely become one of the most rewarding pursuits of your life.

INTRODUCTION: What Makes This Book Special

After reading this Introduction, focus on Chapters **1** & **2**. They contain the essential information you need for succeeding in your upcoming healthy-weight journey.

THIS *INTRODUCTION* contains five parts:

1 – The Core Concept
2 – How This Book is Organized
3 – How This Book Came About
4 – Who Can Benefit from This Book
5 – The Salient Distinguishing Factor

The Core Concept

This book rides on a core concept. That concept is *success action*. Here's how we're using the term.

Success Action:
An action that contributes to creating a certain desired life-enhancing situation

As pertains to this book, the "certain desired life-enhancing situation" is *weight success*. So, what exactly do we mean by weight success? **Weight Success** is: *Living most or all of one's days in one's desired healthy-weight range <u>and</u> deriving benefits, enjoyment, and fulfillment from it.*

You'll be creating weight success by applying a certain success methodology. Applying this methodology will automatically result in success drivers being installed into your weight success pursuit. This, in turn, will result in you succeeding at living the rest of your life in your desired healthy-weight range <u>and</u> deriving benefits, enjoyment, and fulfillment from it.

How This Book is Organized

Contained in this publication is a plethora of useful information. It's made that way to provide maximum bang for your book-buying buck. But you don't need to read it all to succeed at achieving lifelong weight control and healthy-weight living. For that, you only need to read and apply the information in **Chapters One** and **Two**. Every-

thing else is optional backup resource, located in Section B, which you can use as needed.

This book contains five sections: A, B, C, D, E.

SECTION A (p. 16) consists of Chapters 1 and 2. Einstein once said: "If you can't explain it simply, you don't understand it well enough." Chapter 1 presents the essence of this book explained in less than 400 words. From it you will gain introduction to the success methodology presented herein. Then, for fuller detail and insight, proceed to Chapter 2.

Chapter 2 reveals why some people succeed at weight control and others do not. In reading it you will learn of the essential key to more easily creating healthy-weight living. I dub it *Weight Success Secret*. You'll also learn of the powerful new methodology for succeeding at achieving weight control and lifelong healthy-weight living, called *Weight Success Method*™ — or *"the Method"* for short.

SECTION B (p. 70) is for those who want to go beyond the basics. It's for those who want to have all the helpful tactics and information they can get, to make their weight success journey as easy and successful as possible. This section contains over twenty chapters. These chapters provide a plenitude of unique information and insights into the pursuit of weight control and healthy-weight living. If you happen to be a person who likes to dig deep and grasp the big picture, you'll likely find these chapters beneficial and fascinating.

SECTION C (p. 182) lays out a practical plan by which a nation could create universal healthy-weight living among its citizenry.

SECTION D (p. 187) is a Glossary of terms pertaining to weight success and healthy-weight living. When you're not sure what a term means, go to the Glossary.

SECTION E (p. 195) is a handy subject Index — great for finding the location of a bit of information you might be seeking.

How This Book Came About

In case you might like to know, here's how this book and the Weight Success Method came about.

It was summer of '79. For several years I had been grappling with weight gain. My two chief weapons were "one-week diets" and "watching what I ate." Both were annoying — neither effective. Then I decided that exercise might be my salvation. So in July 1979 at age 35 I took up bicycling. I figured it would enable me to eat as much as I wanted without gaining weight. And, for many years it did, *as long as* I was logging over a hundred biking miles a week at vigorous speed.

But then, around 2000 something happened. I was 56 years old, and the happy scenario of eating as much as I liked and burning up these calories with vigorous cycling was no longer working. Two things caused this situation. First, at age 56 I had less muscle mass than at age 35, which resulted in burning fewer calories during biking. Second, I was biking fewer miles and at a slower speed at 56 than at 35, which further resulted in burning fewer calories.

So in 2000 I discovered, to my horror, that I was now gaining weight in spite of bicycling. I was back into the same bad situation I was in in 1979. I was gaining weight and had no easy antidote for it. It was a bummer. But it triggered one of the most gratifying discoveries of my life: the discovery of a method for maintaining my weight exactly where I want it to be *without* pain, hassle, and yo-yo dieting ... and, if necessary, without exercise.

I initially dubbed it "Weight Freedom Method" and later called it "Healthy-weight Method." Finally I adopted the name *Weight Success Method*. And how has this method worked out? Fantastically well! By applying the Method *since 2007* I've been maintaining my weight in my healthy-weight range for nearly every day since. And, most importantly, it has happened easily and enjoyably — and has also brought personal epiphanies and fulfillment.

> If you'd like to know exactly *why* the Method is enjoyable, go to the *Why the Weight Success Method is Enjoyable* chapter, page **123.**

Now, I know some people think the reason I'm living in my healthy-weight range is my body automatically maintains itself at that weight. But that's incorrect. I'm just like everyone else. My body doesn't perform such an incredible feat. I know for a fact it will readily gain at least a pound a week if I let it. For this to happen all I need do is eat just a little more food, or a few more calories per day. If I did that, my body would gain at least a pound a week and in 30 months weigh over 300 pounds.

In short, the Weight Success Method works, and because it does I wrote this book you're now reading. And, how long has it been working? On the bulletin board next to my desk hangs a reminder note. Below is the note for January 1, 2019. It indicates **12** years of living in my healthy-weight range. The number gets updated annually with a new reminder note each New Year's Eve. Believe me, it's a *great* way to kick off each year.

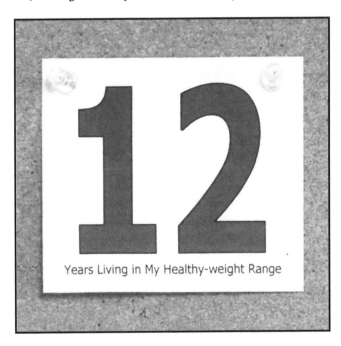

Years Living in My Healthy-weight Range

I see the note every day. I get a good feeling from it every day. As of 2019 I've achieved these many years of healthy-weight living by doing the Weight Success Method. Now here's the main point: *If I can do it, you can do it.* There's nothing special about me. I'm convinced what's working for me will work for you, too.

Who Can Benefit from This Book

You can benefit from the Weight Success Method presented in this book in any of four ways. First, if you've lost weight and are now at your desired weight and want to *easily stay* that way, apply the Weight Success Method and you'll make the weight loss stick for life.

Second, if you're presently in the process of losing weight and you want to do it more *easily* and *enjoyably,* do the Method in combination with the dietary program you're now pursuing and losing weight will become easier and more enjoyable.

Third, if you've never been overweight and you want to ensure you easily stay *non*-overweight the rest of your life, start doing the Method and you'll easily prevent yourself from ever becoming overweight and, thereby, live in your healthy-weight range the rest of your life.

Fourth, if you're overweight and you want to (a) reduce your weight to your desired healthy-weight range and then (b) live in your healthy-weight range the rest of your life, do the Method and it'll happen — and most likely it'll happen more easily and enjoyably than you ever imagined.

The Salient Distinguishing Factor

In the world of dieting and weight control this book stands apart from others. It's because of a certain key distinguishing factor. What most distinguishes this book from all others is:

> This book pursues weight control — a.k.a. healthy-weight living — with a
> ## Success
> ## Methodology

We define *success methodology* as: an action plan that pertains to a certain type of pursuit and consists of specific actions that, when performed by a person, causes a maximal number of success drivers to be included in that pursuit, thereby

resulting in easiest possible creation of the desired situation or outcome associated with the pursuit.

This book presents a success methodology for creating weight success. Or, expressed in detail, it presents a success methodology for living most or all of the rest of your days in your desired healthy-weight range while also deriving benefits, enjoyment, and fulfillment from it. This methodology is what distinguishes this publication from all others.

As previously stated, the name of the success methodology is *Weight Success Method*. You will be acquiring more information on it, and also on success drivers, in upcoming Chapters 1 and 2.

Some people might refer to this book as a "diet book." But that would be an inaccurate description. It's not a diet book; it's a Weight Success Empowerment Book. Meaning, it's a book that empowers people to succeed at achieving weight success by giving them an effective methodology that, when applied, results in the inclusion of success drivers into their weight success pursuit — which, in turn, results in them succeeding at living most or all of the rest of their days in their desired healthy-weight range <u>and</u> deriving benefits, enjoyment, and fulfillment from it.

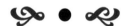

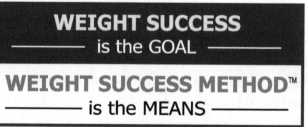

WEIGHT SUCCESS
—— is the GOAL ——

WEIGHT SUCCESS METHOD™
—— is the MEANS ——

Goal+Means+<u>Action</u>=WEIGHT SUCCESS™

WEIGHT SUCCESS = Living most or all of one's days in one's desired healthy-weight range AND deriving benefits, enjoyment, and fulfillment from it.

Most persons who aren't pursuing healthy-weight living are doing so because they're holding an <u>erroneous conception</u> of healthy-weight living. This book changes that situation. It provides an easy, empowering, breakthrough methodology for creating lifelong healthy-weight living. It's called

Weight Success Method.

—

To learn of this Method and how to apply it, all you need do is read Chapters **1** and **2**. Reading this entire book isn't required. Chapters 3–27 are optional backup resources, located in Section B. So to begin, focus on Section A - Chapters **1** and **2**.

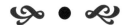

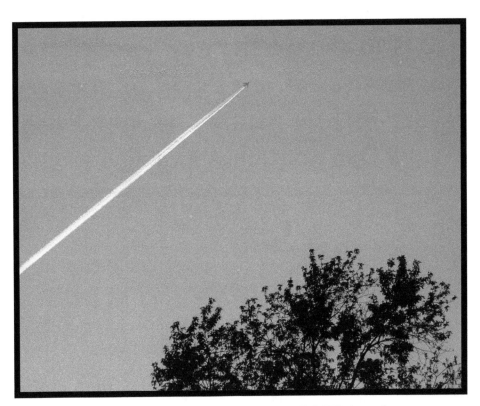

We've taxied the tarmac, now *TAKEOFF* time has come.

SECTION A:
THE ESSENTIAL INFORMATION

THIS SECTION A contains two chapters.

Chapter 1 — titled *This Book in Less than 400 Words* — presents the essence of this book in micro form.

Chapter 2 — titled *Weight Success Method* — discloses the secret, or essential key, to more easily succeeding at achieving weight success for the rest of your life. Then this chapter provides the powerful new weight management methodology called Weight Success Method — a.k.a. *the Method* for short. My experience has led me to conclude that it's the <u>easiest</u> way there is to achieve weight success. And, it typically takes *less than* eight minutes of dedicated time per day to do.

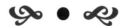

Most people think the first step to healthy-weight living is to change the way one eats. Actually, the first step is to change the way one THINKS — or how one conceives of one's <u>self</u>, of one's <u>mind</u>, of one's <u>life</u>, and of **how healthy-weight living works**. (This Section **A** explains.)

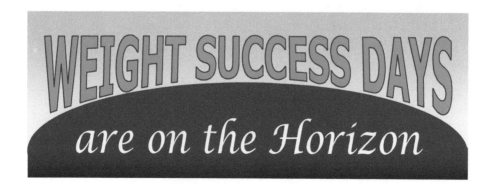

CHAPTER 1: This Book in Less than 400 Words

RECENTLY I came upon a form of literature called micro-fiction. One definition calls it "a story presented in 400 words or less." It got me to thinking, if there's micro-fiction why not micro-*non*-fiction: a piece of non-fiction literature, or a methodology, presented in 400 words or less. So, here's the essence of this book, and the essence of the Method described in Chapter 2, presented in less than 400 words. It's titled *Weight Success Actions are It!*

Weight Success Actions are It!

An action that contributes to you creating weight success we call a *Weight Success Action.* To create lifelong weight success, do Weight Success Actions *every day.* This is the secret to lifelong healthy-weight living. To accomplish it, do these actions — which are the key Weight Success Actions.

FIRST, do these ten *Startup Actions.*

1. Realize that the *real cause* of overweightness is the act of consuming more calories than what your body is metabolizing (p. 35).
2. Identify your desired healthy-weight *range* (p. 36).
3. Identify your desired weight success *benefits* (p. 36).
4. Make weight success a *mandatory* feature of your life (p. 36).
5. Hold the desire and belief that weight success *will* happen and happen *easily* (p. 37).
6. Make your *top* eating priority to be healthy-weight calorie consumption (p. 39).
7. Adopt a bona fide dietary program that fits *you* (p. 40).
8. Set up a *fail-proof* reminder mechanism (p. 41).
9. Obtain a *good* scale (p. 41).
10. Commit to doing *Weight Success Actions* every day (p. 42).

SECOND, after doing the ten Startup Actions, do these five *Daily Actions* each day (which typically takes <u>less than</u> **8** minutes of dedicated time per day).

1. Correctly weigh yourself each day (p. 44).
2A. Each time your daily weight reading is a <u>desired</u> reading, praise yourself (p. 45),
    - OR -
2B. Whenever your daily weight reading is an <u>undesired</u> reading, enact immediate corrective action (p. 48).
3. Each day, direct your mind — including subconscious mind — to act on your eating directions, and also visualize one of your weight success benefits (p. 50).
4. Each day, say your Healthy-weight Goal at least 25 times (p. 54).
5. Each time you eat, apply guided eating (p. 56).

The ten Startup Actions and five Daily Actions constitute a success methodology called *Weight Success Method™.* Doing this method results in you creating weight success — or living most or all of the rest of your days in your desired healthy-weight range <u>and</u> deriving benefits, enjoyment, and fulfillment from it. Lastly, when you seek more in-depth information or an answer to a question, find it in Section B: Optional Backup Resources (p. 70).

* * *

> Now that you know the essence of this book, as expressed in micro form, proceed on to Chapter 2 for greater insight into the powerful Weight Success Method. It's your key to easier lifelong healthy-weight living. And, it typically can be done with <u>less than</u> **8** minutes of dedicated time per day.

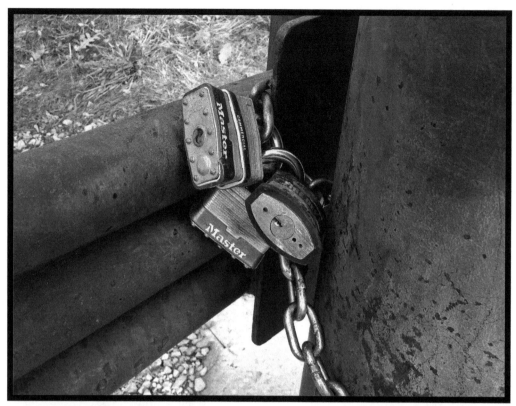

For many people, weight success looks like a multi-padlocked steel gate —
to which they don't have the key. But there <u>is</u> a key to it.
It's the Weight Success Method disclosed in Chapter 2.

The essence of that key can be depicted in a single sentence. We call it the
Weight Success Secret, and it's disclosed in the upcoming pages.

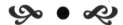

Weight Success is: Living most or all of one's days in one's desired healthy-weight range <u>and</u> deriving benefits, enjoyment, and fulfillment from it. The easiest way to create Weight Success is the **Weight Success Method** — first do the ten Startup Actions and then do the five Daily Actions each day for the rest of your life. By doing this, Weight Success will be <u>YOURS</u>. So ... *read on.*

CHAPTER 2: Weight Success Method

THIS CHAPTER 2 consists of eleven parts (a–k):

Parts (a) through (f) present the foundational concepts of the Weight Success Method. Parts (g) and (h) *describe* the Method. Parts (i) through (k) present follow-up discussion. All subsequent chapters are Optional Additional Resources, located in Section B (p. 70) of this book.

(a) Six Weight Journey Scenarios

A **FIRST STEP** to succeeding at weight control and healthy-weight living is to know the main ways people live their life as pertains to weight management. In modern society most persons live out their life in one of these — or a variation of one of these — six weight journey scenarios. Which one will you live?

Scenario 1: Luck-out — The person effortlessly spends their entire life living at their healthy weight. Their metabolism and rate of calorie consumption are perfectly matched for life. It's a *rare* lucky coincidence.

Scenario 2: Oblivious — At some point the person begins gaining weight. This weight gain is slow but unceasing. It's so slow the person seldom notices the change from month to month. So they never apply a serious preventive measure ... which results in slow, unceasing weight gain for life.

Scenario 3: Fail and Quit — At some point the person begins gaining weight. Eventually they decide to "do something about it." This leads them to pursue "weight control." It takes the form of either (a) an exercise program or (b) a dieting program. Sooner or later, the program "fails" them or they tire of it, so they quit it. They never seriously try again ... which results in weight gain for life.

Scenario 4: Yo-yo — At some point the person begins gaining weight. So they go on a diet. This results in them losing weight. After achieving their weight loss goal they celebrate and go back to "normal living." But the lost weight returns. Still, they're persistent. So, again they go on a diet — and again they lose weight and again it returns. They repeat this process multiple times in their life. We call it yo-yo dieting or yo-yo life.

Scenario 5: Weight Success Action — At some point the person begins gaining weight. They decide to do something about it. So they undertake an exercise program. And, for a while it "works," or at least "helps out." But eventually they realize that the only lasting solution is to manage their eating. So they enact a diet and take their weight down to their healthy weight. Then they make one of the most impacting decisions of their life. They decide that living the rest of their life at their healthy weight is a *mandatory* feature of their life.

This decision causes them to pursue weight control in a different way than most do. Intentionally or non-intentionally, knowingly or not, they begin doing weight success actions <u>every day</u>. And, because they're doing this *they create healthy-weight living for most or all of the rest of the days of their life.*

> **TWO KEY DEFINITIONS:** (1) A *success action* is an action that contributes to creating a certain desired life-enhancing situation. ~ (2) A <u>weight</u> *success action* is an action that contributes to creating weight success, or contributes to living the rest of one's life in one's desired healthy-weight range <u>and</u> deriving benefits, enjoyment, and fulfillment from it. (Keep this definition in mind.)

Scenario 6: Anorexia — At some point the person begins gaining weight. One day they look in a mirror and what they think they see horrifies them, even if they're only slightly overweight. They decide they must lose weight so they won't "be fat." So they reduce food intake and lose weight. But every time they look in a mirror they see only a "fat person," even when they're no longer overweight. So they keep eating less and losing more weight, until they die! What causes this? Astounding as it is, their mindset — or beliefs and views — is what causes them to perform the actions that result in the tragic outcome of scenario 6! In short, it's because of this dynamic:

Mindset → Actions → Outcome

| Mindset | causes → | Actions | causes → | Outcome |

Now here's the key point. *Mindset* is also what causes people to perform the actions that result in scenarios 2, 3, and 4 ... and *mindset* is also what causes them to perform the actions that result in scenario **5.** Please keep this in mind.

(b) The Secret Discovered

RESEARCH TELLS US that about **90** percent of the times when people lose weight they eventually gain it back. Numerous sources substantiate this number. Here, for example, is one such source:

https://healthblog.uofmhealth.org/health-management/weighing-facts-tough-truth-about-weight-loss

So, for every 100 persons who have lost weight and succeeded at achieving a certain desired weight, at least 90 of them have *failed* at maintaining that desired weight. This is a sad situation, indeed. It's a situation that forces a seminal question: WHY is it that, as of year 2020, at least *90 percent* of the people who set out to achieve lifelong weight control eventually fail at it, and only ten percent succeed at it?

For several decades now researchers have been seeking to uncover the factors that have been causing this situation. For easy reference I call these factors *fat-promoting factors.* They are factors that promote overeating and/or weight gain, or that make it easier for a person to overeat and/or gain weight. These researchers have been looking

everywhere and have come up with an amazing compilation of fat-promoting factors.

Several years ago I decided to make myself knowledgeable of these sinister forces. So in December 2015 I conducted some Internet research. I compiled a list of the factors that weight scientists and researchers have "discovered" are a "cause" of overeating and/or weight gain. Here it is.

As of December 2015, here's what researchers have identified as a "cause" of overeating and fat gain: genes, hormones, heredity, body chemistry, brain function, gender, age, menopause, lifestyle, too slow rate of metabolism, expanded appetite or food cravings, decreased smoking, anxiety, stress, depression, lack of sleep, lack of fiber, lack of fatty acids, eating at the wrong time, skipping breakfast, eating foods in the wrong sequence, eating too fast, eating foods derived from grains, eating foods containing "hidden carbs," low-fat foods, salt, sugar, artificial sweeteners, potato chips, food advertising, fast-food restaurants, availability of packaged foods made with too much sugar, artificial additives in food, low cost of food due to agricultural innovation, taste buds insensitivity, too little exercise, working night shifts, unhealthy friends and family, glamorization of overweight-ness, criticism of overweightness, hearing people talk about body weight, thinking you're overweight, too many plus-sized models, yo-yo dieting, age and weight of your mother when you were born, level of carbon monoxide in the atmosphere, indoor temperature too high, lack of air conditioning during hot months, living near a noisy highway or railway or airline flight path, doing repeated decision-making at work, environmental factors that promote eating, endocrine disrupting chemicals such as bisphenol A and phthalates, environmental chemicals such as flame retardants, types of bacteria in your intestine, increasing abundance of food in modern society, certain viruses such as adenoviruses, and certain drugs such as medications that treat depression, heartburn, diabetes, inflammation, allergies, hypothyroidism, hypertension, contraception, and mental illness. Yes, every one has been cited as a factor causing overeating or overweightness.

And, amazingly, the list keeps growing! As previously stated, the above array of fat-promoting factors is current as of *December 2015*. It's much larger as of the date you're reading this, because since 2015 the obsessive quest to "discover" new scapegoat fat-promoting factors has been surging onward.

Not surprisingly, this "science of fat-promoting factors" is super-seductive. When I first encountered it it seemed like some of these factors pertained to me. It seemed like they might be the cause of my overeating and weight gain. Finally, I realized that this "discovering fat-promoting factors craze" is creating one of the craziest, most harmful national delusions in history. It's the *"I can't control my weight"* delusion. This is a *very* dangerous thing. It's dangerous because it leads to the copout conclusion "There's no point in me even trying."

So, don't be sucked into the growing fat-promoting factors movement. Don't let the media hype that publicizes it make you believe you don't control your destiny when it comes to healthy-weight living. Because, you *do* control it.

Sure, some of these fat-promoting factors might promote overeating and make it easier to gain weight. But not a one *causes* a person to overeat or be overweight. Overeating and overweightness are caused by one thing only: overperformance of a certain 3-action process, the process of opening our mouth, inserting food into our mouth, and swallowing the food — a process that happens to be *totally controllable* by each of us. Our failure to recognize and act on this truth is a main factor preventing our succeeding at creating healthy-weight living.

So, we now return to our starting question: Why is it, as of 2020, that 90 percent of the people who set out to achieve lifelong weight control eventually fail at it, and only ten percent succeed at it?

After much thought I finally realized what's happening. It has little or nothing to do with fat-promoting factors. Rather, the ten percent who are succeeding at lifelong weight control are pursuing weight control in a *different way* than the ninety percent who are failing at it. Specifically, those who are <u>succeeding</u> at weight control *are doing weight success actions every day*. Those who are <u>failing</u> at weight control are <u>not</u> doing weight success actions every day <u>or</u> are not doing enough weight success actions every day.

So, what exactly is a weight success action? Again, a *weight success action* is an action that contributes to creating weight success. And, *weight success* is: Living most or all of one's days in one's desired healthy-weight range <u>and</u> deriving benefits, enjoyment, and fulfillment from it.

One of the purposes of this book is to set forth a host of potent weight success actions, which we'll be doing in the rest of this Chapter 2 and in the chapters of Section B. But at this point you might like some specifics. So here are some specific actions that are weight success actions: the ten Startup Actions (p. 35) of the Weight Success Method, the five Daily Actions (p. 44) of the Method, the actions described in the Weight Success Benefits Directive (p. 52), and any action prescribed in the chapters of Section B (p. 70).

Now, distilled to simplest form, here's the key to succeeding at creating lifelong weight success. I've dubbed it Weight Success Secret, for short.

The Weight Success Secret is:
To succeed at lifelong healthy-weight living, *do <u>Weight Success Actions</u> every day.*

By doing Weight Success Actions every day you create Weight Success Days — that is, days that contribute to creating weight success. So, how does one create Weight Success Actions? *Enact a success methodology that, when performed each day, installs success drivers into your daily weight success pursuit.*

Interestingly, this dynamic — the process of daily enacting a success methodology that installs success drivers into a particular pursuit — is the basic dynamic by which success is achieved in virtually every type of significant human endeavor. (Note: This dynamic can happen knowingly <u>or</u> non-knowingly, deliberately <u>or</u> by accident.) Pertaining to the pursuit of weight success, it's my opinion that the most effective success methodology is the Weight Success Method. So, what exactly is (a) a success methodology and (b) a success driver? We answer those two questions in the next sections.

Your weight success journey isn't a month-long, or year-long, or lifelong journey; it's a perpetually repeated **one-day** journey — a one-day journey involving doing weight success actions that day. By repeating this process day after day you become a healthy-weight winner for thousands of days, otherwise known as a lifetime. <u>That's how lifelong weight success is created.</u>

(c) Success Methodology

As previously defined, a *success methodology* is an action plan that pertains to a certain pursuit and consists of specific actions that, when performed by a person, causes a maximal number of success drivers to be included in that pursuit, thereby resulting in easiest possible creation of the desired situation or outcome associated with the pursuit. In this book, the particular success methodology we're talking about is the ***Weight Success Method.***

Moving on, we define *success driver* as: a condition or activity that, when present, increases the likelihood of a person succeeding at a certain pursuit — or, more specifically, increases the likelihood of a person performing actions that foster creation of a certain desired situation or outcome associated with a pursuit.

So, we now describe the anatomy of an effective success methodology.

Two Types of Actions

A success methodology comprises two types of actions: (1) STARTUP actions and (2) DAILY actions.

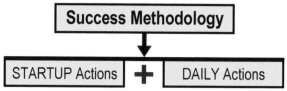

As the term is used here, a *startup action* is an action that's performed at the startup of a particular pursuit. Each startup action installs at least one vital success driver into the pursuit. As pertains to the pursuit of healthy-weight living, there are ten startup actions (p. **35**).

A *daily action* is an action that's performed every day for the duration of a particular pursuit. Each daily action installs into that pursuit one or more vital success drivers. In some pursuits, such as the pursuit of weight success, for example, the duration of the pursuit is "the rest of one's life." As pertains to the Weight Success Method, there are five daily actions (p. **44**).

Two Types of DAILY Actions

For maximal effect a success methodology should include two types of daily actions: (1) goal-realization actions and (2) mind-motivation actions.

A *goal-realization action* is a daily action that leads to attainment or realization of the desired situation or goal associated with a certain pursuit. As regards your weight success pursuit, the actions involved in performing your preferred dietary program (described in Startup Action 7, page 40) are the main goal-realization actions of your weight success journey.

A *mind-motivation action* is a daily action that motivates a person to perform goal-realization actions. Why are mind-motivation actions included in a success methodology? It's because many success pursuits are derailed not because a person doesn't know the actions needed for realizing a particular goal but, rather, because they fail to keep their mind focused and motivated on performing these goal-realization actions each day. In short, mind-motivation actions keep a person focused on performing goal-realization actions.

So, to recap, in your weight success journey the main *goal-realization actions* are those actions involved in performing your chosen dietary program, as described in Startup Action 7 (p. **40**), and the main *mind-motivation actions* are the five Daily Actions of the Weight Success Method, which begins on page **44**.

By now a question has probably come up: How much time is involved in doing the five daily actions of the Weight Success Method? Amazingly, it's very little. It typically takes *less than* eight minutes of dedicated time per day.

(d) Success Drivers

As previously defined, a *success driver* is a condition or activity that, when present, increases the likelihood of a person succeeding at a certain pursuit — or, more specifically, increases the likelihood of a person performing actions that foster creation of a certain desired situation or outcome associated with the pursuit.

So, when success drivers are present, success at a pursuit usually happens — and often happens more easily and enjoyably than what one expects. Conversely, when success drivers are absent, success usually doesn't happen or if it does happen it involves inordinate time and effort. So ...

Success Drivers → Success at a Pursuit
<u>No</u> Success Drivers → <u>No</u> Success

Which means, by installing success drivers into a significant personal pursuit we make each day be a Success Day — that is, a day that contributes to creating a certain desired life-enhancing situation. That's the essential dynamic by which success is created in every significant pursuit — including the pursuit of lifelong healthy-weight living. In infographic form the dynamic looks like this.

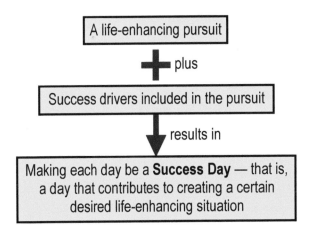

Now we examine success drivers.

Success Drivers for Succeeding at Creating Weight Success

There are 19 main success drivers in the pursuit of weight success. They're the drivers I regard as being most effective for creating success in almost any significant personal pursuit, including the pursuit of weight control and healthy-weight living. The more drivers that are included, the more easily one achieves the desired outcome or goal. Here are those 19 main success drivers.

1 – Achievement goal
2 – Failure cause awareness
3 – Goal-achieving mindset
4 – Enjoyment of process
5 – Motivating reason
6 – Mandate decision
7 – Feedback system
8 – Reminder system
9 – Goal-achieving knowledge
10 – Essential Success Actions
11 – Desire
12 – Focus
13 – Self-communication
14 – Progress tracking and response
15 – Self-reinforcement
16 – Setback surmounting
17 – Persistence
18 – Goal-achieving relationships
19 – Whole-mind involvement

Now, this long list might look daunting. But don't be put off by its length or seeming complexity. Installing these success drivers into your weight success journey is *easy* to do <u>if</u> you take the right approach. This right approach is the success methodology we call *Weight Success Method*. Doing the ten Startup Actions (p. **35**) of the Method helps install Success Drivers #1–9 into your weight success pursuit. Doing the five Daily Actions (p. **44**) helps install Success Drivers #10–19 into your weight success pursuit.

Doing the five daily actions typically takes *less than* eight minutes of dedicated time per day. But before getting into the Weight Success Method we first provide a brief description of the 19 success drivers. (If later you happen to seek a fuller description, go to the *Success Drivers in Depth* chapter, page **137**.)

Success Driver 1:
ACHIEVEMENT GOAL

This driver involves identifying a desired ultimate outcome pertaining to a particular pursuit.

We call this desired ultimate outcome *achievement goal*. As pertains to one's weight success pursuit, the Achievement Goal is: *To be the person of your healthy weight and be healthy, happy, and doing great.* (Note: Your *healthy weight* is every weight in your desired healthy-weight range.) We call this your Healthy-weight Goal.

More on healthy-weight goal comes in *Daily Action 4* (p. **54**).

Success Driver 2:
FAILURE CAUSE AWARENESS

This driver involves recognizing the root activity or factor that causes setback — and perhaps failure — in a particular pursuit.

In a weight success pursuit, the root activity that causes setback and failure is overeating — that is, consuming more calories than what one's body is metabolizing, or "burning up," each day.

More on failure cause awareness comes in *Startup Action 1* (p. **35**).

Success Driver 3:
GOAL-ACHIEVING MINDSET

This driver involves holding a mindset of goal-promoting views and beliefs, and acting as-if these views and beliefs are a true depiction of reality. Remember this:

Mindset → Actions → Outcome

| Mindset | causes | Actions | causes | Outcome |

More on weight success mindset comes in *Startup Action 5* (p. **37**).

Success Driver 4:
ENJOYMENT OF PROCESS

This driver involves identifying or creating a process, or set of actions, by which daily enjoyment is derived from daily pursuit and progressive accomplishment of the Achievement Goal.

When you find the activity involved in achieving a goal to be fun, enjoyable, or otherwise gratifying to do, it makes it easier for you to accomplish the goal because you automatically put more time, focus, and energy into the process. So, as much as feasible you should strive to make the goal-achieving process of healthy-weight living to be fun, enjoyable, and/or gratifying. Yes, it *is* possible to do. Applying the Weight Success Method helps make it happen.

If later you should seek to know exactly how this happens, go to the *Why the Weight Success Method is Enjoyable* chapter (p. **123**).

Success Driver 5:
MOTIVATING REASON

This driver involves identifying the main reason or reasons for pursuing the Achievement Goal.

As pertains to your weight success pursuit, the "main reasons" you have for doing it are the benefits you gain from living in your healthy-weight range. We call these benefits *weight success benefits*.

More on weight success benefits comes in *Startup Action 3* (p. **36**).

Success Driver 6:
MANDATE DECISION

This driver involves deciding that accomplishment of the Achievement Goal is a *mandatory* feature of one's life.

As pertains to your weight success pursuit, you must make the firm decision that living at your healthy weight is a <u>non</u>-optional, <u>will</u>-do, <u>must</u>-have aspect of your existence. You must make this decision and commit to realizing it. Why? Because, if you don't you'll almost certainly fail at creating lifelong healthy-weight living.

> More on mandate decision comes in *Startup Action 4* (p. **36**).

Success Driver 7:
FEEDBACK DECISION

This driver involves identifying or creating a way of measuring daily performance pertaining to realization of the Achievement Goal.

As pertains to your weight success pursuit, the most powerful daily feedback system you can employ is: *daily weighing with an accurate bathroom scale.*

> More on feedback, reinforcement, and correction comes in *Daily Action 1* (p. **44**), *Daily Action 2A* (p. **45**), and *Daily Action 2B* (p. **48**).

Success Driver 8:
REMINDER SYSTEM

This driver involves installing a failproof reminder system.

This is critical for weight success. Why? Because, failure to *remember* to do what one should be doing is a major cause of project failure.

> More on failproof reminder system comes in *Startup Action 8* (p. **41**).

Success Driver 9:
GOAL-ACHIEVING KNOWLEDGE

This driver involves acquiring knowledge vital to achievement of the Achievement Goal.

As pertains to creating weight success, the main goal-achieving knowledge you'll need is contained in this book. So, the way you acquire vital goal-achieving knowledge for healthy-weight living is: Read this book (especially Chapter 2).

Success Driver 10:
ESSENTIAL SUCCESS ACTIONS

This driver involves making sure that the essential success actions are done each day.

Some success actions are "helpful to do." Others are "critical to do every day" — meaning, if they're not done, the likelihood of achieving the Achievement Goal is greatly diminished. We call them *essential success actions*. It's imperative that you do the essential success actions every day.

What are the essential success actions in your weight success journey? They include Daily Actions 1–5 of the Weight Success Method (p. **44**).

Doing essential success actions performs two vital functions. First, it maintains your *daily focus and motivation*. Second, it creates ongoing *daily progress* toward goal achievement. It's worth noting that doing essential success actions each day is at the core of virtually every successful significant personal pursuit.

So, *every day* for the rest of your life do the <u>essential success actions</u> aimed at achieving the goal of lifelong healthy-weight living. That is, every day do the five Daily Actions of the Weight Success Method.

> ## Doing
> ## Weight Success Actions
> ## every day is the Way to
> ## Lifelong Weight Success

Success Driver 11:
DESIRE

This driver involves holding strong daily desire for realizing the Achievement Goal.

It also involves each day fueling this desire by calling to mind the reason for (or benefits to be derived from) goal achievement. Typically, the bigger the goal, the more desire is needed for accomplishing it. Other terms for "desire" are passion, eagerness, determination.

As pertains to your weight success pursuit, to succeed at realizing your Healthy-weight Goal you need to hold *strong daily desire* for its accomplishment. A main way one does this is by staying focused on the benefits — a.k.a. weight success benefits.

Daily Actions 2, 3, and *4* are designed to increase one's desire for healthy-weight living and its benefits. Also, the *Weight Success Benefits in Detail* chapter (p. **80**) explains in depth. Reading this is recommended.

Success Driver 12:
FOCUS

This driver involves each day focusing on the Achievement Goal.

Or, put another way, it involves each day thinking about, talking about, pursuing, and/or deriving enjoyment from the accomplishment or progressive realization of the goal.

The more time you spend focusing on, or paying attention to, a particular goal, the more importance your subconscious mind attaches to that goal. And, the more importance your subconscious mind attaches to the goal, the more it acts to create thoughts and feelings that steer you toward accomplishment of the goal.

So, you must spend time each day *focusing* on the ongoing realization of your healthy-weight goal. A main purpose of doing the Weight Success Method is to cause this daily focusing to happen.

For more on focus, go to the "Cue Type #2: Conscious Mind Focus" section (p. **134**).

Success Driver 13:
SELF-COMMUNICATION

This driver involves sending goal-promoting communications to one's self each day.

Communications you send to your self we call *self-communications*. They are communications you send to your mind — including your subconscious mind. Goal-promoting self-communications trigger your mind to create thoughts and feelings that make goal achievement happen, or happen more easily.

If later you should seek more on this, go to the *Why the Weight Success Method Gets Your Whole Mind Involved* chapter, page **129**. ~ Specifically, go to the "Cue Type #1: Deliberate Communication" section, p. **132**.

Success Driver 14:
PROGRESS TRACKING AND RESPONSE

This driver involves tracking one's daily performance and providing immediate positive response.

For tracking progress one needs feedback. *Feedback* is information that depicts past performance. When the feedback depicts *desired* past performance — a.k.a. progress — you deliver immediate self-reinforcement. When the feedback depicts *undesired* past performance you initiate immediate corrective action. Each is a positive response that expedites goal achievement. Also, for progress tracking to be optimally useful it must be timely. Meaning, for example, daily progress tracking (a.k.a. daily feedback) is usually more useful than, say, weekly progress tracking. In your weight success pursuit, the weight number you get from Daily Action 1 (daily weighing) is the most useful tracking feedback in your weight success journey.

For other examples of progress measuring tools, go to the *Handy Extra Tools* chapter (p. **174**).

Success Driver 15: SELF-REINFORCEMENT

This driver involves delivering reinforcement to one's self after daily progress happens, and telling oneself to keep up the good work.

The act of giving someone something they like as a response or consequence for performing a certain action is known as *reinforcement* — a.k.a. positive reinforcement. When that "someone" is our self, or our mind, we call it *self-reinforcement*. When you deliver self-reinforcement, or appreciation and praise, to your mind — including your subconscious mind — after it assists with creating a certain desired performance it motivates your mind to continue providing that assistance. In short, desired performance followed by reinforcement creates more desired performance.

More on reinforcement comes in *Daily Action 2A* (p. **45**)

Success Driver 16: SETBACK SURMOUNTING

This driver involves holding a productive perspective whenever there's a setback, and also enacting immediate corrective action and converting the setback into a progress action.

In every major endeavor — including the pursuit of weight success — setbacks occur. Success depends on the response to these setbacks. When one responds in a counterproductive way it results in turmoil, frustration, and defeat. But when one responds in a productive way it results in (a) learning from the setback and (b) converting it into a progress action.

More on setback surmounting comes in *Daily Action 2B* (p. **48**) and also in the *Setback Reversal Made Easier* chapter (p. **88**).

Success Driver 17: PERSISTENCE

This driver involves persistently pursuing the Achievement Goal, and pressing on in spite of challenges, setbacks, or discouragement.

The realization that unceasing persistence is a key to achieving any major goal isn't new; it has been around for decades. Many names have been applied to it. Examples include: persistence, perseverance, determination, tenacity, doggedness, pressing on, stick-to-it-ness, gutting-it-out, and grit.

So, as pertains to your weight success journey, *don't give up*. Instead, each day press on toward continued accomplishment of your worthy healthy-weight goal. Which means, never cease doing essential Weight Success Actions every day. If you do this, which includes doing the Weight Success Method, you *will* achieve your goal.

Success Driver 18: GOAL-ACHIEVING RELATIONSHIPS

This driver involves discovering and building relationships that encourage and assist one in accomplishing the Achievement Goal.

This success driver does not apply to every type of pursuit. But it can be made to apply to most. And, when it is applied it can be powerful.

As pertains to your weight success pursuit, productive relationships can expedite achievement of your healthy-weight goal at least two ways. First, they can be a means for sustaining motivation and productive mindset during the pursuit of the goal. Second, they can be a means for obtaining valuable assistance — such as, advice, know-how, key resources — that can be helpful in expediting goal achievement. This assistance can be obtained from productive interaction with people and also God.

Lastly, it's important to note that one might find it helpful to downplay relationships or interactions that run counter to achievement of one's life-enhancing goals.

For more on relationships, see the *Escaping Schaden-freude* chapter (p. **121**) and the relationships section (p. **160**) of the *How the Weight Success Method Enhances Your Life Journey* chapter, and the *Three Steps to Getting Input from God* section (p. **117**).

Success Driver **19**:
WHOLE-MIND INVOLVEMENT

This driver involves having one's whole mind — that is, both conscious <u>and</u> subconscious mind — involved each day in the pursuit of the Achievement Goal.

As pertains to your weight success pursuit, when your whole mind is involved each day in the pursuit of your healthy-weight goal something powerful happens. It results in your subconscious mind stepping up and assisting with achievement of that goal. Your subconscious mind does this by creating thoughts and feelings that make you more effective at (a) surmounting obstacles and (b) obtaining what you need for goal achievement. Which means, the more involved your subconscious mind is in the achievement of your healthy-weight goal, the easier the achievement of that goal becomes.

When your subconscious mind is working to steer you toward achieving your healthy-weight goal it creates goal-promoting thoughts and feelings that guide you toward living in your healthy-weight range. This results in you doing right eating and weight control. Conversely, when your subconscious mind *isn't* involved in steering you toward achieving your healthy-weight goal it *doesn't* create goal-promoting thoughts and feelings. This results in overeating and weight gain. And, when you cycle between the two — that is, your subconscious mind is involved for a period, stops being involved for a period, starts again, stops again — you lose weight, gain weight, lose weight, gain weight — a condition called yo-yo dieting.

I call all that *The Whole-mind Dynamic of Healthy-weight Living*. Most people are unaware of this dynamic. So, they don't realize that a main success driver of healthy-weight living is:

Have your WHOLE mind — that is, both conscious <u>and</u> subconscious mind — involved *each day* in the pursuit of living in your healthy-weight range.

As an infographic, the Whole-mind Dynamic looks like this.

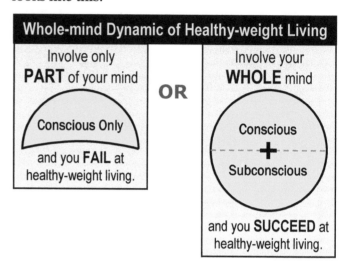

So, be sure to include this Success Driver 19 in your weight success journey.

Does the thought of "having your whole mind involved each day in the pursuit of living in your healthy-weight range" seem complex or hard to do? Well, good news, it's not. It's actually simple and easy **if** you do this: <u>Apply the Weight Success Method</u>. Doing the five daily actions of the Weight Success Method (p. 44) typically takes less than eight minutes a day. Yet it causes you to have your WHOLE mind involved *each day* in the pursuit of healthy-weight living. And this, in turn, *greatly* increases the likelihood of you succeeding at creating healthy-weight living for life.

For more on whole mind involvement, go to the *Why the Weight Success Method Gets Your Whole Mind Involved* chapter (p. **129**).

Societal Impact of the Whole Mind Dynamic

Here's how the Whole-mind Dynamic applies society-wide. Those few people who are living in their healthy-weight range likely have their *whole* mind — or both conscious <u>and</u> subconscious mind — involved each day in the pursuit of healthy-weight living. This involvement of their whole mind comes about either intentionally or non-intentionally or both.

Conversely, most of those people who are continuing to live <u>above</u> their healthy-weight range do *not* have their whole mind involved each day in the pursuit of healthy-weight living.

What's more, those who lost weight *while* dieting and then gained the weight back *after* the dieting had their whole mind involved *during* the dieting but stopped having their whole mind involved *after* the dieting!

Trying to achieve your biggest goals using only the "conscious half" of your mind is like trying to take a canoe trip using "half a canoe." Applying the Weight Success Method is the easiest way to ensure you're taking your whole canoe on your weight success journey.

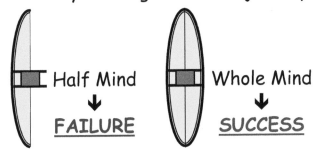

Present View of Weight Management

So, how does our society view weight management? Many people view it as primarily a dietary process. Others view it as mainly an exercise process. Still others view it as basically a medical procedures process. But fundamentally it's a *daily success-creation* process. When we don't approach it as that, weight-control failure usually results.

Now, I know that diet, exercise, and medical procedures can play a part in creating weight management success for many people. But for maximum effect we must apply these factors *in conjunction with* most or all of the 19 success drivers, not as a substitute for them. So, as a standalone solution — diet, exercise, and medical procedures are less than fully effective, but as part of a daily success-creation process, each can sometimes be helpful.

SUMMATION to This Point

A review of key concepts to this point would prove worthwhile. So here's a summary of ten key concepts thus far.

1 — Persons succeed at weight management when they're doing Weight Success Actions *every day*. When they're not doing daily Weight Success Actions they usually fail at weight management.

2 — This explains why many persons succeed at weight reduction and then 9 out of 10 eventually fail at weight maintenance. It's because while pursuing weight reduction they're doing Weight Success Actions every day, and then later when "pursuing" weight maintenance they're no longer doing Weight Success Actions every day, or are doing fewer Weight Success Actions. The result is: They succeed at weight reduction, then after that fail at weight maintenance.

3 — This leads us to an underlying dynamic, which we dub Weight Success Secret. The Secret is: To succeed at lifelong healthy-weight living, *do Weight Success Actions <u>every day</u>*. By doing this we create continual Weight Success Days — that is, continual days that contribute to creating weight success.

4 — So a pivotal question arises: For any given pursuit, such as healthy-weight living, how does one go about doing success actions every day? The answer: *The person enacts a success methodology that, when performed each day, installs success drivers into that pursuit.* Interestingly, this dynamic — the process of implementing a success methodology that installs success drivers into a particular pursuit — is the basic dynamic by which success is achieved in virtually every form of significant life-enhancing endeavor. It might be done knowingly <u>or</u> non-knowingly, deliberately <u>or</u> by accident.

We define *success methodology* as an action plan that pertains to a certain pursuit and consists of specific actions that, when performed by a person, causes a maximal number of success drivers to be included in that pursuit, thereby resulting in easiest possible creation of the desired situation or outcome associated with the pursuit.

In this book, the particular success methodology set forth for creating weight success is the *Weight Success Method*. Doing the Method typically takes <u>less than</u> **8** minutes of dedicated time per day.

5 — We define *success driver* as a condition or activity that, when present, increases the likelihood of a person succeeding at a certain pursuit — or, more specifically, increases the likelihood of a person performing *daily actions* that foster creation of a certain desired situation or outcome associated with a pursuit. As pertains to the pursuit of weight success, we identified 19 success drivers. The ten Startup Actions help install Success Drivers #1–9. The five Daily Actions help install Success Drivers #10–19.

6 — The more success drivers that are present in a pursuit, the greater the likelihood that a person will succeed at the pursuit. Conversely, the fewer success drivers that are present, the lesser the likelihood that a person will succeed. So, by installing success drivers into a particular pursuit — including the pursuit of weight success — we gain the ability to create the desired situation or outcome associated with that pursuit.

7 — So, how does one easily include these success drivers into their weight success pursuit? They apply the Weight Success Method.

8 — After using the Weight Success Method and living in my healthy-weight range for *more than* ten years now (as of the start of writing this book), I've had an epiphany: The Weight Success Method is the easiest way to apply the Weight Success Secret. Which means, it's the easiest way to do Weight Success Actions *every day* — which results in creating continual Weight Success Days.

Note: If you'd like to have fifteen more reasons for using the Weight Success Method, go to the *Attributes of an Ideal Weight Management Program* chapter (p. **73**).

9 — So here's my best suggestion. To apply the Weight Success Secret and, thereby, create healthy-weight living for life, *do the Weight Success Method*. That is, first do the ten Startup Actions (p. **35**), then do the five Daily Actions (p. **44**) every day thereafter. Doing the five daily actions typically takes *less than* eight minutes of dedicated time per day. That's a very small amount of time. So, there's no valid reason why it can't be done.

10 — By doing the Weight Success Method you will automatically include most or all of the 19 success drivers into your weight success journey, which will result in you succeeding at more easily creating lifelong weight success. In infographic form it looks like this.

10 Startup Actions **+ 5** Daily Actions of the Weight Success Method

results in

Success Drivers Being Included in Your Weight Success Pursuit

results in

Creating lifelong Weight Success — a.k.a. Lifelong Healthy-weight Living <u>and</u> Benefits

So, what the above ten points boil down to is this. When pursuing weight <u>reduction</u> do the Weight Success Method. This causes success drivers to be included in your weight *reduction* pursuit. After achieving your desired weight and going into weight <u>maintenance</u>, continue doing the Weight Success Method. This causes success drivers to be included in your weight *maintenance* pursuit.

Why the Weight Success Method Works

There's a reason the Weight Success Method is so effective in creating weight success. It's because of a certain universal dynamic, which is this: *The desired outcome of nearly every significant personal pursuit is realized by having <u>success drivers</u> present in that pursuit.* When success drivers are present, the likelihood of creating the desired outcome of the pursuit is maximized and, as a result, it's almost always achieved. Summed up in one sentence: The Weight Success Method works because it installs success drivers into your weight success pursuit.

Here's an infographic depicting that dynamic.

Pursuit + Success drivers →
Creating desired outcome of the pursuit

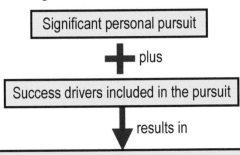

So all you need do now is finish reading this Chapter 2 and then apply the Weight Success Method *each day* for the rest of your life. Remember: Doing the five daily actions of the Weight Success Method typically takes *less than* eight minutes of dedicated time per day.

(e) Success Killers

THE PRIOR section described 19 vital elements for succeeding at weight control and healthy-weight living. We dubbed them *success drivers*.

This section introduces the flip-side of the weight success coin. It lists 21 conditions that can cause a person to fail at weight control and healthy-weight living or, at least, cause that person to experience needless hassle and difficulty in pursuing weight control. We dub these 21 conditions *success killers*. They're coming up next.

Now here's a key point. Many success killers are "the opposite" of success drivers. Which means, a success killer comes in when the corresponding success driver is absent. Finally, keep in mind that the easiest, most effective way to install success drivers is via the Weight Success Method.

> Should you desire fuller explanation, go to the *Success Drivers and Success Killers in Depth* chapter (p. **137**).

The top 21 success killers to <u>avoid</u> are:

1. Believing that there's "no problem" in being "a little bit" overweight.
2. Believing that there are factors beyond one's control that are making one overeat and gain weight — or, put another way, believing that weight control is impossible.
3. Believing that weight control is hard to do.
4. Believing that doing weight control is unpleasant and enjoyment-robbing.
5. Believing that lack of exercise causes over-weightness and that more exercise is a requirement for creating weight control and weight success.
6. Not realizing that the first step to weight-control success is *mindset* change.
7. Not identifying one's desired healthy-weight range.
8. Not deciding that healthy-weight living is *mandatory*.
9. Not identifying one's weight success benefits.
10. Not identifying healthy-weight calorie consumption as the top priority of eating.
11. Not adopting a dietary program that fits *you*.
12. Not remembering to do what one needs to be doing every day.
13. Not getting daily feedback derived from daily weighing.
14. Not keeping healthy-weight living a *top* priority.
15. Not responding to setbacks in a productive way.
16. Not ignoring negative comments by others.
17. Not doing guided eating most of the time.
18. Not viewing healthy-weight maintenance as a noteworthy accomplishment.
19. Not involving one's whole mind each day.
20. Not applying a *daily* success methodology for pursuing healthy-weight living.
    > Tip: The easiest, most effective weight success methodology I know is the Weight Success Method.
21. Not doing Weight Success Actions *every* day, or not making each day a Weight Success Day.

(f) Intro to the Weight Success Method

TO INTRODUCE the Weight Success Method we're going to summarize six foundational concepts of this book, then provide five pointers for maximizing success on your upcoming weight success journey.

Six Foundational Concepts: Summed Up

The weight range that provides greatest likelihood of you living in good health we call your *healthy-weight range.*

Living most or all of your days in your healthy-weight range is a situation we call *healthy-weight living.*

The easiest way to create healthy-weight living is the Weight Success Method. The Weight Success Method is a *success methodology* for achieving weight success. That is, it's an action plan that consists of specific actions that, when performed by a person, causes a maximal number of success drivers to be included in their weight success pursuit, which results in the person creating healthy-weight living and deriving benefits, enjoyment, and fulfillment from it.

A *success driver* is a condition or activity that, when present, increases the likelihood of a person succeeding at a certain pursuit. Doing the Weight Success Method automatically results in the inclusion of success drivers (p. **23**) in one's healthy-weight pursuit.

The Weight Success Method comes in two parts. The first part comprises ten *Startup* Actions (p. 35); the second part comprises five *Daily* Actions (p. 44). The Startup Actions are performed at the beginning of your weight success journey; the Daily Actions are done each day thereafter. Doing all five Daily Actions typically takes *less than* **8** minutes of dedicated time per day. Plus, doing them is easy.

The Weight Success Method activates a certain key dynamic that we call Weight Success Secret. Expressed in a single sentence, the Secret is this: To succeed at lifelong healthy-weight living, *do Weight Success Actions every day.* This makes each day be a Weight Success Day. The easiest way to apply the Secret is do the Weight Success Method.

Five Pointers for Maximizing Success on Your Upcoming Weight Success Journey

While on your weight success journey please do the following five things. By doing so you will maximize your effectiveness and success.

Success Pointer 1 — *Focus on Daily Progress Action.* Realize that success in any major pursuit derives from small progress actions performed day after day. (Another term for *progress action* is "step in the right direction.") Further, realize that small daily progress actions can be performed at any chosen time on any given day. Still further, realize that, distilled to its essence, your weight success journey constitutes an endless series of daily progress actions — or "steps in the right direction" — performed day after day for a lifetime. Finally, realize that performing these progress actions can be simple, easy, and enjoyable.

Success Pointer 2 — *Hold a Can-do, Will-do Mindset.* Hold the view and belief — a.k.a. assumption — that you can and will achieve lifelong healthy-weight living. And, also hold and act on the assumption that you'll achieve it *easily,* or at least more easily than you likely ever imagined.

Success Pointer 3 — *Keep in Mind that the Easiest Road to Healthy-weight Living is the Weight Success Method.* Realize that this is because the Weight Success Method is the easiest way to bring success drivers into your weight success pursuit which, in turn, enables creating the desired outcome of the pursuit.

Success Pointer 4 — *Take Advantage of All Available Resources.* Section B (p. **70**) holds a plethora of optional backup resources. More than likely, whenever you have a question or seek more in-depth information or come upon a special problem, the insight and information you need and seek exists within Chapters 3–27. To find it, review the Table of Contents (p. **6**) *and/or* go to the Index (p. **195**) *and/or* check out the Glossary (p. **187**).

Success Pointer 5 — *Adapt, Improvise, Enhance.* As of the start of writing this book I've spent more than twelve years creating, personally testing, modifying, refining, editing, and writing the success methodology I call Weight Success Method. As a result, the ten Startup Actions and the five Daily Actions that constitute this Method are exact procedures. I urge you to put these procedures to the test by applying them specifically and fully. I do this because I'm convinced that if you fully apply these procedures you'll reap rewarding results.

But, very few things in this world are perfectly perfect. No matter how good and complete something is there's usually some way — if only a small way — that it can be modified to be better or more effective. This is especially the case when dealing with a human-applied methodology created for worldwide individual use. This happens because each of the several billion members of humankind is, in at least some small way, unique unto itself.

So in addition to my urging you to exactly, fully apply the prescribed actions of the Weight Success Method I *also* urge you to be open and eager to adapting, improvising, and enhancing any of those actions to your personal situation, should you see a way of doing so. This could maximize the impact of the Method in your weight success journey.

Now, finally, the time has come for you to begin the ten Startup Actions (p. 35) of the Weight Success Method. I believe you'll discover this to be the first step of one of the most rewarding accomplishments of your life: the noble, noteworthy accomplishment known in this book as *weight success* — a.k.a. living most or all of the rest of your days in your desired healthy-weight range <u>and</u> deriving benefits, enjoyment, and fulfillment from it.

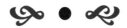

THE WEIGHT SUCCESS SECRET IS THIS:

To succeed at lifelong healthy-weight living, do Weight Success Actions <u>every</u> day. Likely the most powerful Weight Success Actions are the five Daily Actions (p. 44) of the Weight Success Method. Doing these actions installs <u>success drivers</u> into your weight success pursuit. It typically takes <u>less than</u> **8** minutes of dedicated time per day. The result is this activates a certain **Weight Success Dynamic,** shown below.

WEIGHT SUCCESS DYNAMIC

Doing Weight Success METHOD each day	installs	Success DRIVERS into Weight Pursuit	which creates	Experiencing Weight SUCCESS

WEIGHT SUCCESS = Living most or all of one's days in one's desired healthy-weight range <u>and</u> deriving benefits, enjoyment, and fulfillment from it. ~ For description of benefits created by weight success, see Chapter 7 (p. **80**). For description of enjoyment and fulfillment created by doing the Weight Success Method and achieving healthy-weight living, go to Chapter 17 (p. **123**), Chapter 22 (p. **157**), and Chapter 24 (p. **168**). ~ A person who's in process of creating weight success we call a *Weight Winner.*

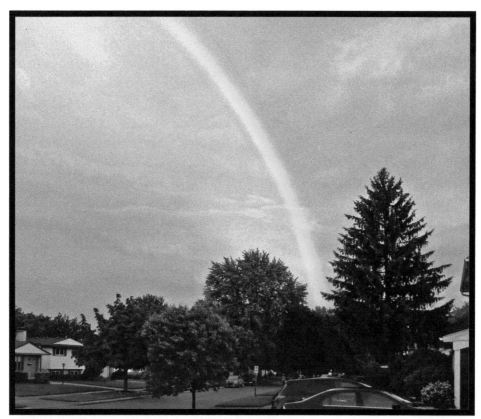

There <u>is</u> a pot of gold at the end of the Healthy-weight Living Rainbow —
it's a basket of Weight Success BENEFITS. The easiest way to capture
these benefits is: Do the Weight Success Method <u>every day</u>.

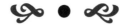

DO
WEIGHT SUCCESS ACTIONS
EVERY DAY.

This is the way weight success is created. Likely, the most effective Weight Success Actions are the actions of the **Weight Success Method.** Doing the Method typically takes <u>less than</u> **8** minutes of dedicated time per day. This installs vital success drivers into your weight success pursuit, which results in you experiencing weight success for life.

(g) Weight Success Method — Part 1: Ten STARTUP Actions

The Weight Success Method comes in two parts: (1) STARTUP Actions and (2) DAILY Actions. This is the FIRST Part. Doing these 10 Startup Actions helps install Success Drivers #1–9 into your Weight Success Pursuit.

DOING THE upcoming ten startup actions lays the foundation for succeeding at lifelong healthy-weight living. It helps you install Success Drivers #1–9 into your weight success journey. You do these ten actions at the beginning. But bear in mind, to create maximal success in your weight success pursuit you must retain the result of these actions, or keep acting upon the decisions made in these actions, throughout your weight success journey — meaning, each day for the rest of your life.

The WEIGHT SUCCESS METHOD begins with these ten Startup Actions:

Action 1: FAILURE CAUSE (p. **35**)

Action 2: WEIGHT RANGE (p. **36**)

Action 3: WEIGHT SUCCESS BENEFITS (p. **36**)

Action 4: MANDATORY FEATURE (p. **36**)

Action 5: MINDSET (p. **37**)

Action 6: EATING APPROACH (p. **39**)

Action 7: DIETARY PROGRAM (p. **40**)

Action 8: REMINDER (p. **41**)

Action 9: SCALE (p. **41**)

Action 10: THE KEY (p. **42**)

The 10 Startup Actions form the foundation upon which lifelong Weight Success is created.

Startup Action **1:** FAILURE CAUSE
Recognize the *real* cause of overweightness.

There's only one real cause of our overweightness. It's *overperformance* of a certain three-action process, the process of:

1 – Opening our mouth;

2 – Inserting a piece of metabolizable calorie-containing food into our mouth; and

3 – Swallowing the piece of food.

We call it the *Open–Insert–Swallow* process — or **O-I-S** process, for short.

Overperformance of this process is the <u>real</u> cause of overeating and weight gain. And, it's the only cause. This process is how we consume more metabolizable calories than what our body is metabolizing, or "burning up," per day, which in turn is what causes us to gain weight. Lastly, recognize that this process is *totally controllable* by each of us.

So ...

Even though much of society refuses to admit it, weight gain and overweightness is created by our actions and, therefore, is controllable by each of us.

OVERPERFORMANCE OF

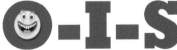

The REAL Cause of Overweightness

> **Definition:** *Overeating* is the act of consuming more calories than what our body is metabolizing, or "burning up," per day.

Startup Action 2: WEIGHT RANGE

Identify a desired healthy-weight *range.*

Instead of using a single pound or kilogram number as your weight target or goal, use a weight *range.* And, make the range wide enough that it's possible — with a reasonable effort — to get *within* the range on most or all of your days. By using a weight range as your goal you have opportunity to be a weight management *success* all or most of the time. This weight range becomes the essence of your Healthy-weight Goal — a.k.a. weight goal or achievement goal.

So ...

For starters, set your ideal weight range span to be six, seven, or eight pounds or, if you weigh in kilos, three or four kilograms. Then, view every number in your healthy-weight range as being a *healthy weight* for you. Which means, whenever your body weight is in your healthy-weight range you're living at your healthy weight, a situation we call *healthy-weight living.* For example, if your weight range were 158–164 pounds, then each day your weight is between 158.0 to 164.9 pounds you would be "at your healthy weight."

For more, go to the *Healthy-weight Range in Detail* chapter (p. **76**). Reading this is recommended.

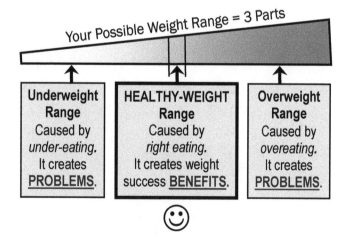

Startup Action 3: BENEFITS

Identify your weight success *benefits.*

Having a good reason for doing something builds our motivation to do it and increases our resoluteness to press on when a setback occurs. As regards the pursuit of weight success, the "good reason" we have for doing it is the benefits we gain from living in our healthy-weight range. We call these benefits *weight success benefits.*

So ...

Identify your weight success benefits. Then reflect on these benefits each day. By doing this it motivates your mind to pursue activities that lead to realizing these benefits, which includes the activity of creating healthy-weight living success. Here's an infographic.

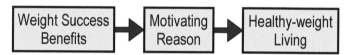

For more, go to the *Weight Success Benefits in Detail* chapter (p. **80**). Reading this is recommended.

Startup Action 4: MANDATORY FEATURE

Decide that healthy-weight living is a *mandatory* feature of your life.

Mandatory feature means: <u>non</u>-optional, <u>will</u>-do, <u>must</u>-have aspect of your existence. Most people who fail to create healthy-weight living have also failed to make the firm decision that living in their healthy-weight range is a mandatory feature of their life. When living in your healthy-weight range *isn't* a mandatory, must-have aspect of your life, you tend to get discouraged or quit whenever a setback arises.

So ...

Decide right now that living in your healthy-weight range is — and will continue to be — a *mandatory* feature of your existence. Then, hold this decision in mind for the rest of your life.

```
┌─────────────────────────────────────┐
│   Startup Action 5: MINDSET         │
├─────────────────────────────────────┤
│   Adopt a weight success mindset.   │
└─────────────────────────────────────┘
```

Startup Action **5**: MINDSET

Adopt a *weight success mindset.*

Our dominant views and beliefs — a.k.a. assumptions — shape our life. They do this by triggering thoughts, feelings, and actions that work to create actual situations that correspond to the imagined situations depicted within our views and beliefs. In doing so, our beliefs affect every aspect of our existence, *including* that aspect called eating and weight management.

Sadly, as pertains to weight management many people hold self-defeating views and beliefs. They believe — or assume — that either (a) they can't succeed at living their desired weight or (b) if they do succeed at it it will involve hardship and suffering. This results in them never even trying to live their desired weight or, if they do try, eventually quitting because they find it to be "hard."

> SIDE NOTE: At this point I must make an admission. I believe *anyone* can (a) succeed at living most or all of their days at their healthy weight and (b) do it easily and enjoyably. I further believe, based on personal experience, that the quickest way to make this happen is by doing the Weight Success Method described in this chapter.

So ...

Realizing the huge impact of our beliefs on our life, what should we be doing? We should be holding views and beliefs that promote creation of the situations we want to have happen — including the situations of (a) controlling our weight and living in our healthy-weight range and (b) doing it *easily.*

As pertains to creating lifelong healthy-weight living, there's a particular mindset — which we call *weight success mindset* — that consists of seven key views and beliefs. Holding this mindset opens the door to the easiest way to create weight control and healthy-weight living. For ease of expression, I'll describe it like a person would express it.

My weight success mindset includes these views and beliefs:

1. Living in my healthy-weight range requires doing Weight Success Actions *every day.*

2. Living in my healthy-weight range is a <u>mandatory</u> feature of my existence — so, living outside that range is a <u>non-option</u>.

3. Living in my healthy-weight range provides me many great benefits.

4. I possess the power to make it happen — that is, I possess the power to (a) direct my eating, (b) direct my thoughts and feelings as pertains to eating, (c) live in my healthy-weight range *and* do it easily, and (d) surmount any fat-promoting factor I might encounter.

5. For me, right eating is more enjoyable and rewarding than wrong eating.

6. For me, correct calorie consumption is more important and rewarding than maximization of eating pleasure.

7. I view every challenge and setback in my weight success journey as a stepping stone to greater personal progress and future healthy-weight living, and not as a millstone holding me back from future success.

Holding a mindset of the above seven elements maximizes your effectiveness at achieving weight control and healthy-weight living. Here's why. Your mind — including your subconscious mind — creates thoughts and feelings that align with your major beliefs. Which is to say, your mind seldom operates in contradiction to your major views and beliefs, or outside the boundaries defined by those views and beliefs. So you should make sure all your eating- and weight-related mindset elements are ones that promote right eating and living in your healthy-weight range, and that none of them promote wrong eating or living outside your healthy-weight range. The above seven elements have maximal impact on creating the types of thoughts and feelings that promote right eating and healthy-weight living. So, they should be part of your "eating and weight management mindset."

Now here's a main point: <u>Doing the Weight Success Method assists you with installing these mindset elements into your mind</u>.

So, ask yourself this question: *How do I want my weight success journey to be?* Do I want it to be tough? (It can be that.) Or, do I want it to be easy? (It can be that, too.) So decide now how you *want* it to be and *believe* it will be:

Hard	*Easy*
	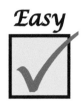

In short, weight management is either: (a) depressing drudgery or (b) uplifting journey. *You* determine, in large part, which it will be by the desires and the beliefs you hold in your mind. So, hold the desire and the belief that it will be *easy* ... or, at least, way easier than you ever imagined it could be. In short, succeeding at creating healthy-weight living depends, to a large extent, on you *believing* and *acting as-if* you possess the power to make it happen.

How Believing and Acting As-if Work

Here's why believing and acting as-if are important. The act of *believing* that your mind is *in the process* of performing certain actions is one of the most powerful tools there is for succeeding at healthy-weight living (and other pursuits, as well). So, each day hold the belief that your mind — including your subconscious mind — is acting on what you want it to be doing. This includes holding the belief that your mind is pursuing the healthy-weight living goal you want it to be pursuing.

Also ... Act As-if

Along with believing, act as-if. That is, conduct your thinking, feelings, and actions in accordance with the belief that your mind — including subconscious mind — is right then in the process of listening to and taking action on everything you're telling it. When you do this it motivates your mind to create the types of thoughts and feelings you desire to have, which in this case are thoughts and feelings

that steer you toward right eating and healthy-weight living.

But, what should you do if you find it hard to muster the belief that your mind is acting on what you're telling it? Again, the answer is: Act as-if. To do this, *you totally pretend you believe.* That is, you role-play that your mind — including subconscious mind — is right then in the process of doing what you're telling it to do. And, in doing this role-play you hold in mind the thoughts and feelings that would be present within your mind if your mind was, in fact, right then doing what you're telling it to do.

Perhaps all this seems a bit odd. But do it anyhow — it works. It triggers your mind to produce the thoughts and feelings you desire to have — in this case, thoughts and feelings that guide you to lifelong healthy-weight living.

Acting as-if is one of the most powerful tools there is for making healthy-weight living happen. So, hold in mind the assumption that you have the wherewithal to easily make healthy-weight living happen, then conduct your thinking, feelings, and actions in accordance with that assumption.

> **Definition of Acting As-if:** *Acting as-if* is the act of holding in mind an assumption that a particular situation presently exists or is in the process of coming about, and then conducting one's thinking, feelings, and actions in accordance with that assumption.

Your thoughts and feelings determine your eating actions, your eating actions determine your weight. You <u>do</u> have the power to create and hold healthy-weight-promoting thoughts and feelings each day.

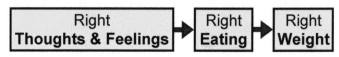

There are two main approaches to eating: (1) *pleasure* priority approach and (2) *healthy-weight* priority approach. Each exerts a powerful impact: one negatively, the other positively.

With the **PLEASURE priority approach** the main goal is *eating pleasure maximization.* Unfortunately, this leads to over-performing the Open–Insert–Swallow process. Which, in turn, results in overeating and weight gain. As such, the pleasure priority approach makes weight control *very* hard to do. This is a main factor causing people to struggle with creating healthy-weight living.

> **Definition of Overeating:** *Overeating* is the act of consuming a greater number of calories than what your body is metabolizing, or "burning up," per day.

But with the **HEALTHY-WEIGHT priority approach** the main goal is: eating an amount of calories that leads to healthy-weight living — otherwise called *healthy-weight calorie consumption.* This approach results in performing the Open–Insert–Swallow process to a proper extent. As such, it leads to non-overeating and living in one's desired weight range.

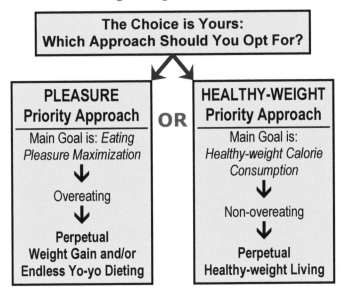

The Choice is Yours: Which Approach Should You Opt For?

PLEASURE Priority Approach	OR	HEALTHY-WEIGHT Priority Approach
Main Goal is: *Eating Pleasure Maximization* ↓ Overeating ↓ **Perpetual Weight Gain and/or Endless Yo-yo Dieting**		Main Goal is: *Healthy-weight Calorie Consumption* ↓ Non-overeating ↓ **Perpetual Healthy-weight Living**

Regrettably, most persons opt for the pleasure priority approach. This dooms them to regular overeating and weight gain which, in turn, makes it nearly impossible for them to succeed at living their life in their healthy-weight range.

So ...

Avoid the pleasure priority approach to eating and embrace the healthy-weight priority approach.

Now, at this point you might be thinking: "Yes, healthy-weight calorie consumption looks like the smart option, but pleasure maximization is the *fun* option, so that's for me." That's how most people view it, which is why most people are endlessly gaining weight. But they're mistaken about the healthy-weight priority approach. It can be enjoyable and gratifying too, when applied a certain way. That "certain way" I call *right eating.*

Right Eating – Way to Healthy-weight Living

With **Right Eating** there are three priorities:

1 – Healthy-weight calorie consumption (top priority)
2 – Proper nutrition
3 – Eating enjoyment.

Each priority has a purpose. The purpose of priority #1 is healthy-weight living, or living your life in your healthy-weight range. The purpose of priority #2 is having an optimally healthy body. The purpose of priority #3 is eating enjoyment derived while pursuing priorities #1 and #2. So, right eating promotes healthy-weight living, optimally healthy body, and eating enjoyment.

Also, each priority is achieved a certain way. You achieve priority #1 by eating a certain *amount* of food — specifically, an amount that results in healthy-weight calorie consumption. I call this amount **right amount.**

You achieve priority #2 by eating certain *types* of food — that is, types that promote good health. I call these types of food *right types,* or **right foods.**

You achieve priority #3 by performing priorities #1 and #2 with a certain enjoyment-creating approach — specifically, an approach that results in savoring and appreciating the flavors of right foods in right amounts. I call this *right eating enjoyment* or, simply, **right enjoyment.**

So here's my one-sentence definition of right eating. **Right Eating** is: Eating right foods in right amounts, and in a way that creates right eating enjoyment. Here's an infographic.

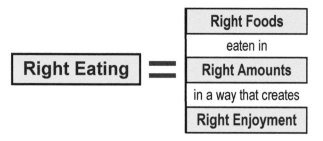

At this point you might be thinking, "Okay, sounds good, but how do I create right eating enjoyment?" Here are four guidelines for it.

> **Definition:** A *healthy-weight-promoting food* is a food that promotes creation of healthy-weight living.

Guidelines for Creating Right Eating Enjoyment

1. Create lower-calorie, *healthy-weight-promoting foods* that are <u>tasty</u> and <u>satisfying</u>.

2. Prepare *healthy-weight-promoting foods* that are easy to consume in right amounts and also <u>more satisfying</u>.

3. Eat *healthy-weight-promoting foods* in a way that maximizes <u>eating pleasure</u> derived from these foods.

4. Condition your mind to enjoy *healthy-weight-promoting foods* and to not enjoy overweight-promoting foods. This might sound hard to do, but actually it's fairly easy once you get into it.

> For more on this subject, go to page **102**.

Conclusion. Keep in mind the concept of Right Eating. It's a key concept to avoiding overeating and achieving easier healthy-weight living. And remember, of the three factors that constitute right eating, *healthy-weight calorie consumption* is the top priority. So, always remember, the <u>real</u> cause of overweightness is:

OVERPERFORMANCE OF

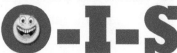

(Overperformance of Open–Insert–Swallow Process)

Almost every successful weight management pursuit involves a preferred dietary program. I define *preferred dietary program* as a set of eating guidelines and eating practices you prefer to follow and which, when followed, cause you to realize good health and healthy-weight living. When you don't have a dietary program that you're applying it increases the chances of you eventually straying "off course" and ending up gaining back the weight you once lost. Another name for preferred dietary program is preferred eating strategy.

Virtually any bona fide dietary program will work when it's *fully* applied. But most people never apply a program fully. Why? Because they're pursuing a program that doesn't fit their personal preferences, needs, and lifestyle. This results in them finding the program to be hard to do, so they quit.

So …

Find the program that best fits your personal preferences, needs, and lifestyle. This is a key to dietary program success because the program that best fits you is the one you're most apt to apply fully. In short: full application = works fully; partial application = works partially or not at all. And, the program you're most apt to apply fully is the one that best fits you and your situation.

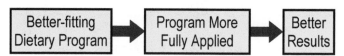

If you don't yet have a preferred dietary program you have a choice. It can be one of the bona fide established programs already on the market *or* it can be a program of your own design. Go whichever way will produce the best results for you.

> Your **preferred dietary program** is a set of eating guidelines and eating practices you prefer to follow and which, when followed, cause you to realize good health and healthy-weight living.
> For a preferred dietary program you have two choices:

Do one of the established bona fide dietary programs on the market.	**OR**	Do a dietary program of your own design (but make sure it's healthy).

If you're thinking about traveling the design-it-yourself road, be sure to apply the basic principles of nutrition so you avoid inadvertently adopting a harmful eating practice.

> For info and ideas on creating a self-designed program, go to the *Author's Approach to Eating* chapter (p. **94**).

A dietary program can be a straight-forward plan — such as eating a certain number of calories per day. Or, it can be a detailed program involving eating certain specific foods in certain amounts. Or, it can be any other nutritionally sound program involving a certain focus, procedures, or guidelines.

So, your objective should be either to find or to design the dietary program that *best fits you*. Hold this thought in mind: Somewhere in the world is a dietary program with "your name on it." If you desire to have it and believe you can get it, you'll eventually find it or create it.

Also, bear in mind you can change your dietary program any time you find a better one. So it's not required that you obtain the "perfect dietary program" before beginning weight management. You can start with an "acceptable" or "best available" program and then later, when you discover a better program, you can switch.

To conclude, it goes without saying that whatever dietary program you follow should be one that doesn't harm your health or create a potential medical problem. And, it could be a good idea to consult with your physician before adopting any new dietary program or making a major change in eating practices.

Startup Action **8**: REMINDER

Install a *failproof* reminder mechanism.

A main factor causing many people to fail at creating healthy-weight living is the act of *forgetting* to apply their weight management program.

So ...

Set up a *failproof* reminder mechanism that will remind you each day to apply the Weight Success Method. Make reminder messages to yourself. Then place these messages where you'll see them every day. Possibilities include: (a) in your bedroom, (b) on the refrigerator, (c) in your wallet or purse, (d) in your car, (e) on your computer, and (f) on your exercise equipment. Plus, put digital messages on your computer screen, smartphone, and other devices. Do whatever it takes to create a failproof reminder system. Here's an example reminder message.

> # Weight Success Method
> Do it every day. Takes less than **8** minutes.
> **1** – Weighing
> **2** – Reinforcement or Correction
> **3** – Benefits Directive
> **4** – Goal Statement
> **5** – Guided Eating
> (plus Daily Exercise Activity)

> For more on setting up a reminder system, go to the *Setting Up a Fail-proof Reminder System* section, on page **180**.

Startup Action **9**: SCALE

Obtain a *good* scale.

The biggest irony in the world of weight control is this. The dreaded bathroom scale, which most folks despise and ignore, is the very thing that has the power to set them free. Here's why. When properly used, as described in Daily Action 1 of the Weight Success Method (p. 44), it delivers timely feedback that enables a person to take control of their weight management destiny.

So ...

If you don't already have one, get a consistently accurate scale. Then make your scale a favorite tool and a friend.

> (For more on scales, go to the *Weighing and Scale Info* chapter, page **82** — reading this is recommended.)

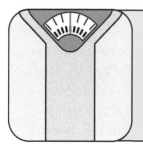

SECRET: Properly used, any good bathroom scale is the most powerful tool on the planet for creating healthy-weight living. Sadly, this fact is one of our "world's best-kept secrets."

Startup Action **10:** THE KEY
Commit to doing *Weight Success Actions* <u>every</u> day.

Never forget: The #1 reason why we fail at creating healthy-weight living is we fail to do Weight Success Actions every day.

So ...

Apply the success methodology we call *Weight Success Method*. The five Daily Actions in the Method are some of the most powerful Weight Success Actions a person can do. Doing the Method installs most or all of 19 success drivers (p. 23) into your weight success journey which, in turn, results in making most or all of your days be a Weight Success Day.

Summed up, all this results in the Weight Success Dynamic shown below.

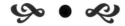

WEIGHT SUCCESS DYNAMIC

Doing Weight Success METHOD each day	installs	Success DRIVERS into Weight Pursuit	which creates	Experiencing Weight SUCCESS

WEIGHT SUCCESS = Living most or all of one's days in one's desired healthy-weight range <u>and</u> deriving benefits, enjoyment, and fulfillment from it. ~ For description of benefits created by weight success, see Chapter 7 (p. **80**). For description of enjoyment and fulfillment created by doing the Weight Success Method and achieving healthy-weight living, go to Chapter 17 (p. **123**), Chapter 22 (p. **157**), and Chapter 24 (p. **168**). ~ A person who's in process of creating weight success we call a *Weight Winner*.

> ## Doing
> ## Weight Success Actions
> ## every day is the Way to
> ## Lifelong Weight Success

REMEMBER: The key to succeeding at healthy-weight living is: Do Weight Success Actions <u>every day</u>. The 10 Startup Actions are your launch pad in this process. They help install Success Drivers **#1–9** into your weight success pursuit.

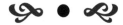

KNOW THIS AND NEVER FORGET IT.
You possess the capability to create healthy-weight living for life, and also the capability to create it **EASILY**. The five Daily Actions are your next step. They help install Success Drivers **#10–19** into your weight success pursuit.

WEIGHT SUCCESS
—— is the GOAL ——

WEIGHT SUCCESS METHOD™
—— is the MEANS ——

Goal+Means+<u>Action</u>=WEIGHT SUCCESS™

WEIGHT SUCCESS = Living most or all of one's days
in one's desired healthy-weight range AND
deriving benefits, enjoyment, and
fulfillment from it.

(h) Weight Success Method — Part 2: Five DAILY Actions

The Weight Success Method comes in two parts: (1) STARTUP Actions and (2) DAILY Actions. This is the SECOND Part. Doing these five Daily Actions helps install Success Drivers **#10–19** into your Weight Success Pursuit.

AFTER COMPLETING the ten Startup Actions you begin the five Daily Actions (Part 2 of the Method). In doing so, bear in mind three things about these five actions.

1. They're *easy* to do.
2. In total, they typically take *less than* eight minutes of dedicated time per day.
3. They can be *combined* with any bona fide dietary program of your choice, including one of your own design.

The five DAILY ACTIONS of the Weight Success Method are:

1 – WEIGHING (p. **44**)

2A – REINFORCEMENT (p. **45**)
— OR —
2B – CORRECTION (p. **48**)

3 – BENEFITS DIRECTIVE (p. **50**)

4 – GOAL STATEMENT (p. **54**)

5 – GUIDED EATING (p. **56**)

By doing these five Daily Actions each day (and also having done the ten Startup Actions) you go a long way toward installing most or all of the 19 success drivers (p. 23) into your weight success pursuit. This results in you realizing the desired outcome, or goal, of the pursuit. The following pages tell how to do these five Daily Actions.

> ## Doing
> ## Weight Success Actions
> ## every day is the Way to
> ## Lifelong Weight Success

> ### Daily Action **1:** WEIGHING
>
> **Correctly weigh yourself each day (and weigh only once a day).**

This action typically takes <u>less than</u> 30 seconds.

WHY You Do It

Correct daily weighing is the *#1 most important* action for creating healthy-weight living. It's because of three outcomes. First, weighing each day creates *daily focus* on healthy-weight living. Second, it provides *timely feedback* on your prior day's healthy-weight efforts. Third, it enables you to give *immediate positive response* to your daily weight situation. There are two positive responses. When your daily weighing shows a <u>desired</u> weight you respond with reinforcement (Daily Action 2A). When the weighing shows an <u>undesired</u> weight you respond with immediate corrective action (Daily Action 2B). These three outcomes — daily focus, timely feedback, and immediate positive response — make correct daily weighing the #1 most important action in your weight success journey.

HOW to Do It

Create *accurate* weight readings. Your daily weight reading can vary slightly from weighing to weighing due to variables unrelated to fat gain or loss. We call these variables ***extraneous variables.*** Possible extraneous variables include: (a) when you last ate, (b) amount of water retention by your body, (c) amount of urine in your bladder, (d) amount of clothes you have on, (e) type of floor the scale is on, (f) location of the scale on the floor, (g) where you stand on the scale, and (h) where you distribute your body weight on your feet. You should strive to minimize the effect of these variables. To do that apply these eight rules.

Eight Rules for Correct Daily Weighing

Apply these eight rules every time.

1. **Use a good scale.** If possible, use one that's consistently accurate. Use the *same* scale for each weighing.

2. **Weigh at the *same time*,** or within the *same hour*, each day (and only once a day). The best time usually is in the morning prior to breakfast. Call it your Daily Weighing Hour. As an example, my daily weighing hour is 7:00 to 8:00 a.m.

3. **Avoid eating before weighing.** If you must eat soon, eat after the weighing.

4. **Empty your bladder before weighing.**

5. **Weigh yourself with nothing on,** or else with the same weight of clothing every time. (You'll likely find that weighing naked is the easiest way.)

6. **Position the scale on the same spot on the floor.**

7. **Stand on the same spot on the scale.**

8. **Use the same weight distribution on your feet.** It doesn't matter what the weight distribution is as long as it's the same with each weighing.

In short, weigh yourself in a way that accurately measures fat change (or non-change) from day to day. For this, weigh yourself at the *same time,* or in the same hour, and in the *same way* each day. The object is, make the extraneous variables be the same with each weighing. The best time for weighing is most likely in the morning before breakfast. Make it one of the first actions of each day.

Plus, when the final weight reading comes up on the scale, *SAY* that weight number to yourself.

Note on Scales. With many scales if you weigh yourself twice in a row it will give you two slightly different readings. If your scale is one of these, weigh yourself twice in a row at each weigh-in and then go with the *average* of the two numbers. But, if your scale is a consistently accurate one, weigh yourself just once.

For more on scales and weighing, go to the *Weighing and Scale Info* chapter (p. **82**).

SUMMING UP This Daily Action 1

Weigh every day, the same time, the same way, using the Eight Rules for Correct Daily Weighing each time. ~ Do this, and also the other four daily actions of the Weight Success Method, and lifelong healthy-weight living will be *yours*.

REMEMBER: The secret to succeeding at lifelong healthy-weight living is: Do Weight Success Actions <u>every</u> day. You accomplish this by doing the Weight Success Method, which typically takes <u>less than</u> 8 minutes of dedicated time per day. This causes vital *success drivers* to be included in your weight success pursuit.

Daily Action **2A**: REINFORCEMENT
Each time your daily weight reading is a <u>desired</u> reading, respond with self-reinforcement.

This action typically takes <u>less than 40 seconds</u>.

Desired weight readings exist in two forms: (a) readings that come during weight maintenance pursuit and (b) readings that come during weight reduction pursuit. When in weight <u>maintenance</u> pursuit — or striving to maintain a certain weight — any reading that's within your healthy-weight range we call a *desired* weight reading. When in weight <u>reduction</u> pursuit — or striving to lose weight — any reading that's lower than the prior day's weight reading we call a *desired* weight reading.

Each day that you get a desired weight reading you follow up by delivering self-reinforcement to your mind — especially subconscious mind.

WHY You Do It

When your subconscious mind receives reinforcement — that is, an enjoyable or desirable response — for a particular action it performed, it motivates your subconscious mind to repeat that action. In this instance, the action for which your subconscious mind is receiving reinforcement is the act of creating thoughts and feelings that guide you to getting desired weight readings. Because of this dynamic, this Daily Action 2A increases the likelihood of having future desired weight readings.

HOW to Do It

One of the most powerful forms of reinforcement is sincere appreciation and praise. So, each day after your daily weighing, when you've discovered once again that you're living another day in your healthy-weight range, give your mind — that is, your self — praise and appreciation. Tell it you're super happy over the desired weight reading, and that you want it to keep up the good work. And, when delivering this self-communication, do it with exuberance and joy. In short, use your daily weighing each morning as a springboard for creating daily pride, happiness, and inspiration. It's a great way to start a day. I've been doing it for years. It never gets stale.

Recommended Message

To make it easy for you, following is a message I suggest you use for your self-reinforcement (the shaded italic paragraph in the next column). I call it the *Thank You, Keep It Up* message. For the blank line, insert one of these two phrases, whichever applies:

continue living in my healthy-weight range
— OR —
lose more weight.

Insert the first phrase when you're in weight maintenance pursuit, the second one when in weight reduction pursuit.

You deliver the message by speaking either in regular-volume voice or in a whisper — your choice.

Thank you, thank you, thank you, subconscious mind! Thank you for guiding me to

_____.
*I really, truly appreciate you doing this. Keep it up. Keep on creating daily <u>thoughts</u> and <u>feelings</u> that guide me to consuming the **types** of food and the **amount** of food that results in me living each day of the rest of my life in my healthy-weight range. I <u>very much</u> want you to do this. And, I believe <u>one hundred percent</u> that you <u>will</u> do it. Great work, subconscious mind! Keep it up. Thank you, thank you, thank you!*

The above Thank-you, Keep It Up message includes the phrase "subconscious mind." It's there to ensure that your subconscious mind focuses on what you're saying, so that it will "hear" the message and then *do it*.

As explained in the Whole Mind Involvement discussion (p. **28**), a main driver of successful healthy-weight living is having your whole mind — that is, both conscious and subconscious mind — involved each day in the pursuit of healthy-weight living.

One of the most effective ways of getting one's subconscious mind involved is direct communication — that is, directly communicating requests, directives, depiction statements, and thank-you messages to it. (This we do in Daily Actions 2A–5.)

For maximal impact, I suggest you address your subconscious mind by a name. It can be any name you like. You can use a person-type name, such as, for example, your first name. And, your subconscious mind will respond to that name as long as it knows you're speaking to it. Also, naming your subconscious mind "Subconscious Mind" is okay, too. Or, if you like, you can use a nickname such as, for example, "Sub-mind" or "Subby Mind" or "Subby." For what it's worth, I use the nickname Subby. Seems like a corny name, I know, but I've used it for years and my subconscious mind has readily responded to it.

Six Actions for an Effective Thank You, Keep It Up Message

To maximize the effect of your Thank You, Keep It Up message, do these six actions when delivering it.

1. **Use a name**: Address your subconscious mind by *a name* — again, the name I use is "Subby," but the name "Subconscious Mind" and other names will work, too.

2. **Be specific**: Describe the *specific* desired action your subconscious mind has performed.

3. **Express appreciation**: Deliver *thanks and appreciation* for having performed the desired action.

4. **Request continuance**: Tell your subconscious mind to *continue performing* the desired action.

5. **Express desire**: Express the continuance request with *strong desire,* or emotional intensity.

6. **Express belief**: Express *firm belief* and also *act as-if* your subconscious mind is right then in the process of doing what you're requesting.

NOTE: The prior Thank You, Keep It Up message (p. **46**) incorporates all six actions — check it out.

The wording for the Thank You, Keep It Up message can vary slightly from weighing to weighing, as you might ad lib. But it mainly embodies the prior italic paragraph on page **46**. TIP: Make a copy of it and keep it where you can easily refer to it.

Deliver the Thank You, Keep It Up message in a way that creates maximum positive impact on your mind. So as you say it, generate a feeling of happiness and joy, joy over having gotten a desired weight reading for yet another day — which means you're either in your healthy-weight range or moving toward it. The more joy you experience and express, the more it motivates your mind — in particular, your subconscious mind — to continue creating desired weight readings.

Also, when delivering the message — and during the rest of your day — *hold the belief* that your mind is right then, at that very moment, *in the process* of performing the actions described in the message. This enhances the impact.

For more information on believing and acting as-if, go to the *How Believing and Acting As-if Work* section in Startup Action 5 (p. **38**). Reading this is *recommended.*

The prior example Thank You, Keep It Up message takes only about 30 seconds to deliver. Yet it's powerful. When reinforcing your subconscious mind there's no such thing as too much thanks and appreciation. So it's okay to include more praise and thanks than what's in the example message. Heap it on — with exuberance.

ADDITIONAL REINFORCEMENT. For more reinforcement for daily good performance, check out "Mind Motivator 6: Goal Reminders" on page **115** in the *Six More Mind Motivators* chapter. An example of a strong visual reminder is the note shown on page 13. It's recommended that you post visual reminders of your healthy-weight goal and of your ongoing realization of that goal. Then view these reminders throughout each day, and especially when doing this Daily Action 2A.

OPTIONAL PRAYER. If you're one who likes prayer, here's one you might use after each weighing.

I thank you, God, for making me to be,
and for the opportunity to become the finest person I'm
*   capable of being,*
and for the opportunity to live in my healthy-weight range,
and for the opportunity to do it easily.
I thank you very, very much.

It's a pithy expression of gratitude. It's also thought-provoking. I've been saying it for years right after delivering the Thank You, Keep It Up message. I find it motivating and uplifting.

SUMMING UP This Daily Action 2A

After each desired weight reading, thank and reinforce your mind — including your subconscious mind — and tell it to keep up the good work. When doing this, include the Thank You, Keep It Up message (p. **46**). Deliver the message using the Six Actions for an Effective Thank You, Keep It Up Message. ~ Do this Daily Action 2A each time you get a desired weight reading, and also do the other four daily actions of the Weight Success Method, and healthy-weight living will be *yours.*

REMEMBER: The secret to succeeding at lifelong healthy-weight living is: Do Weight Success Actions <u>every</u> day. You accomplish this by doing the Weight Success Method, which typically takes <u>less than</u> **8** minutes of dedicated time per day. This causes vital *success drivers* to be included in your weight success pursuit.

Daily Action **2B:** CORRECTION

Whenever your daily weight reading is an <u>undesired</u> reading, respond with immediate corrective action that very day.

So, what's an undesired weight reading?

When in weight <u>maintenance</u> pursuit, any daily weight reading that's outside, or above, your healthy-weight range we call an *undesired* weight reading. And, when in weight <u>reduction</u> pursuit, any daily weight reading that's higher than the prior day's weight reading we call an *undesired* weight reading.

Each time you get an undesired weight reading you should initiate corrective action.

WHY You Do It

Taking immediate corrective action fixes the undesired weight problem within 24 to 48 hours. This puts you instantly back on track to lifelong healthy-weight living and ensures that a small problem doesn't grow into a big one. In short, it *ensures* that your healthy-weight pursuit *never fails*.

The procedure for taking immediate corrective action varies between the two types of weight management pursuits. So, first I describe how to do it in weight maintenance pursuit, and then in weight reduction pursuit.

How to Take Corrective Action When in Weight *MAINTENANCE* Pursuit

To correct, or reverse, an undesired weight reading when in weight maintenance pursuit — or when striving to maintain a certain weight — do these two actions.

First, avoid negative reaction. That is, don't get involved in second-guessing, self-doubt, self-pity, self-blame, guilt, or discouragement. Instead, declare the day to be a *Weight Correction Day*. View this Weight Correction Day as an exciting opportunity to build your personal strength and healthy-weight management expertise. This is *very* important.

Second, enact immediate corrective eating action. For the next 24 or 48 hours eat in a way that corrects the undesired situation in that time. To do this, go into *under-eating* mode. That is, consume fewer calories than what your body will be expending. You can do this with either total fasting or semi-fasting. With total fasting you eat nothing for that period. With semi-fasting you eat just a small amount.

> **Note:** If engaging in under-eating could create a problem or be harmful to you, find out from your doctor what a safe minimal number of daily calories is for you. Then consume that daily amount for the duration of your under-eating period. As always, before adopting any new dietary program or major change in eating practices you should consult with your physician.

If you opt for semi-fasting do this. Pick a "calorie target" — like, say, for example, 600 calories for the day. And then consume only that many calories. Does this seem like it would be hard to do? Well, it's not. Just make the decision to do it and then do it. If you feel that this would be difficult, or might be a burden on you, bear this point in mind.

Correcting a weight-gain situation after it has become big is about a *hundred* times harder than correcting it when it's small, or first crops up. So, eagerly correct the problem *now*. In doing this, don't view a weight correction day as a hardship; view it as an opportunity — an opportunity to save yourself a massive amount of future hardship by expending a miniscule amount of effort and "suffering" today, or for just 24 hours. So, *never* procrastinate on fixing an undesired weight reading. Always do it *that very day*. Typically, going into under-eating mode will bring your body weight back into your healthy-weight range in just 24 to 48 hours.

> For further benefit, do the *setback-reversal process* described in the *Setback Reversal Made Easier* chapter starting at page **88**.

Reminder Note: When your daily weight reading shows a <u>desired</u> weight, you do Action **2A** and not 2B. When it shows an <u>undesired</u> weight you do Action **2B** and not 2A.

Staving Off Hunger Pangs. If you find yourself being nagged by hunger pangs while doing this Action 2B, apply one or more of these three tactics.

Tactic 1: Drink Water. When you feel a hunger pang drink some water. This fills your stomach, which reduces the hunger pang.

Tactic 2: Deliver a Mini-directive. Before drinking the water, deliver this directive to your subconscious mind: "Subconscious mind, after I finish drinking this water, neutralize my hunger pang for the next two hours. I *know* you can do it. I *want* you to do it. I believe one hundred percent that you *will* do it. And, I thank you for doing it."

Tactic 3: Say the Goal Statement. Silently say this healthy-weight goal statement throughout the day, especially whenever you feel a hunger pang.

> "I <u>am</u> the person of my healthy weight.
> I am healthy, happy, and doing great."

In short, whenever a hunger pang arises, focus your mind on your healthy-weight goal.

How to Take Corrective Action When in Weight *REDUCTION* Pursuit

To respond appropriately to an undesired weight reading when in weight reduction pursuit — or striving to lose weight — do these four, or possibly five, actions.

ACTION 1: *Be Real.* ❧ Realize that an undesired weight reading can occur from extraneous variables (listed in Daily Action 1, page **44**). So,

bear in mind that this particular undesired reading might be a result of that. If it is, then the variable that caused today's "weight gain reading" will likely cause a "weight loss reading" tomorrow or the day after, when the variable is working in reverse. Also, make sure you're applying the Eight Rules for Correct Daily Weighing every day (described in Daily Action 1).

ACTION 2: *Avoid Negative Reaction.* ❧ Avoid second-guessing, self-doubt, self-pity, self-blame, guilt, and discouragement. All these are counter-productive. Instead view the undesired weight reading as an opportunity to improve your weight management expertise. This is *very* important.

ACTION 3: *Do Your Full Dietary Program.* ❧ Make sure you're following your weight-loss regimen, or preferred dietary program, completely. If you haven't been, recommit yourself to doing so, then start doing it that very day. <u>Also</u>, make sure you're doing all five daily actions of the Weight Success Method <u>every day</u>.

ACTION 4: *Reverse the Setback.* ❧ If you've gotten an undesired, or weight gain, weight reading <u>three</u> days in a row, do the setback-reversal process described in the *Setback Reversal Made Easier* chapter (p. **88**).

ACTION 5: *If the Above Actions #1–4 Aren't Working, Consider a Change of Dietary Program.* ❧ If you've done the above four actions completely and are still getting too many undesired weight readings, give serious consideration to replacing your present dietary program with another one, one that better fits you and your situation. For more on dietary programs, see Startup Action 7 (p. **40**).

In short, if your weight reduction pursuit is involving too many undesired weight readings it means one or both of two things: (a) you're not fully doing your preferred dietary program and/or (b) you're using the wrong dietary program and you need to switch to one that's better suited to your situation, needs, and preferences. Whichever is the cause, don't procrastinate on putting the corrective action into effect right away. If you have the *right* dietary program for you <u>and</u> you're implementing it *fully* each day, you <u>will</u> lose weight.

SUMMING UP This Daily Action 2B

Whenever you get an undesired weight reading while pursuing weight *maintenance,* (a) hold a positive outlook and (b) take immediate corrective action that very day — that is, immediately bring your weight back into your healthy-weight range, typically within 24 hours. ~ Whenever you get too many undesired weight readings while pursuing weight *reduction,* make sure that (a) you're applying the optimal preferred dietary program for you and (b) you're implementing that program fully each day. ~ Do this Daily Action 2B when it's called for, and lifelong healthy-weight living will be *yours.*

REMEMBER: The secret to succeeding at lifelong healthy-weight living is: Do Weight Success Actions <u>every</u> day. You accomplish this by doing the Weight Success Method, which typically takes <u>less than</u> 8 minutes of dedicated time per day. This causes vital *success drivers* to be included in your weight success pursuit.

```
┌─────────────────────────────────────────┐
│  Daily Action 3: BENEFITS DIRECTIVE      │
├─────────────────────────────────────────┤
│  Each day, read your Weight Success      │
│  Benefits Directive, then visualize one of the │
│  benefits as an accomplished fact.       │
└─────────────────────────────────────────┘
```

This action typically takes *less than* three minutes.

A copy of the Weight Success Benefits Directive is at the end of this Daily Action 3 section, pages **52–53.**

WHY You Do It

Delivering your Weight Success Benefits Directive to your self does three powerful things. First, it describes for your mind — mainly, your subconscious mind — the exact mindset and actions that it should focus on bringing about for creating lifelong healthy-weight living. Second, it instructs your subconscious mind in what it should be doing each time you say your Healthy-weight Goal Statement (Daily Action 4). And, third, it reminds you of your weight success benefits. The result: Delivering the Directive motivates your subconscious mind to each day create the types of thoughts and feelings that lead you to creating lifelong healthy-weight living.

HOW to Set Up the Directive

In the Directive, fill in these blank lines: (a) healthy-weight range, (b) preferred dietary program, and (c) weight success benefits. You'll find the Directive on pages 52–53 (and also at the end of this book, page 205) and also in the Toolkit at: correllconcepts.com/toolkit.pdf

> For more on setting up the Directive, go to the *Detailed Instructions for Weight Success Benefits Directive* chapter (p. **85**). Reading this is recommended.

HOW to Deliver the Directive

When delivering the Directive each day do these four things.

First, do the actions described in the instructions section at the top of the first page.

Second, read the Directive aloud. (Reading aloud is best, but when you can't do that, whisper it to yourself.)

Third, after reading it, pick out one of the more exciting weight success benefits and visualize yourself enjoying it. Visualize for at least 30 seconds.

Fourth, when delivering the Directive — and throughout the rest of your day — *hold the belief* that your subconscious mind is right then, at that very moment, *in the process* of performing the actions described in the Directive. For more information on this, go to the *How Believing and Acting As-if Work* section in Startup Action 5 (p. **38**).

> For greater detail on delivering the Directive for maximal impact, read the *How to Deliver the Weight Success Benefits Directive for Maximal Effect* section (p. **54**).

How to Get Copies of the Directive

Make several copies of the Weight Success Benefits Directive (p. 52–53) for your personal use, and place the copies in spots where it'll be convenient (like, perhaps, a copy in your suitcase).

Also, there's an extra copy at the end of this book (p. 205), in case you'd like to cut it out.

Plus, another way to get copies is go to the free online Toolkit at:

correllconcepts.com/toolkit.pdf

There you'll find a PDF document of the Benefits Directive formatted for printing on 8.5×11-inch paper. If you like, you can print it out two-sided and, thereby, have the entire Directive on a single sheet.

Also, if you'd like to have the Directive in a format that might be handy for keeping on a digital device — computer, tablet, or smartphone — go here: **correllconcepts.com/dir-dig2.pdf** Copy or upload it to your digital device.

SUMMING UP This Daily Action 3

Each day deliver the Weight Success Benefits Directive (which starts on page 52). Deliver it to your subconscious mind, and also visualize one of your weight success benefits. During the day, believe and act as-if your subconscious mind is in the process of performing every instruction you give it. ~ Do this Daily Action 3, and also the other four daily actions of the Weight Success Method, and lifelong healthy-weight living will be *yours*.

REMEMBER: The secret to succeeding at lifelong healthy-weight living is: Do Weight Success Actions <u>every</u> day. You accomplish this by doing the Weight Success Method, which typically takes <u>less than</u> **8** minutes of dedicated time per day. This causes vital *success drivers* to be included in your weight success pursuit.

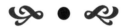

Almost no one enjoys being overweight, but most of us are; almost all of us would like to live non-overweight, but most of us don't. This is the head-scratcher of the 21st century.

Weight Success Benefits Directive

INSTRUCTIONS: Use this Directive for Daily Action 3. ● Where there's a dotted line (...........), say the name you use when speaking of or to your subconscious mind. ● Read this directive aloud <u>and</u> say it with some emotional intensity. (Reading aloud is best, but when you can't do that, whisper it to yourself.) When reading it, **strongly desire** for the actions it describes to be realized. And, **hold the belief** and act as-if what's described in this statement is *in the process of happening.* After reading the list of weight success benefits, for at least 30 seconds **visualize** at least one of the benefits as an accomplished fact. As you go through the day, *continue* believing and acting as-if what's described in this directive is in the process of happening. ● For set-up, insert your healthy-weight range and preferred dietary program into the blanks. For the "pounds–kilos" phrase, draw a line through the word that doesn't apply. List your weight success benefits on the lines at the end. Hint: Use pencil, not pen. Or, type it up and tape it in. (For more, see the Detailed Instructions for Weight Success Benefits Directive chapter, page 85.)

* * *

........................., I want you to do these five very important actions, today and *every* day for the rest of my life.

1 – Guide me to *easily* living in my **healthy-weight range,** which right now is

_____ to _____ pounds–kilos.

2 – Guide me to *fully* doing my **preferred dietary program**, which right now is the

_____ program.

3 – When I say my Healthy-weight Goal Statement while eating, automatically create thoughts and feelings that guide me to Right Eating, that guide me to eating the ***types*** of food and the ***amount*** of food that results in me living in my healthy-weight range.

4 – Whenever I make a decision to stop eating, make the urge to eat *immediately* begin to fade away for that eating session. And, if anytime I happen to accidentally overeat, create an uncomfortable bloated feeling that lasts for a short time.

5 – Whenever I say my Healthy-weight Goal Statement, bring to mind a thought of at least one of my weight success benefits. And, then, create within me a *happy, positive feeling.*

The Weight Success Benefits I gain from living in my healthy-weight range include:

  1. A greater chance of *living healthier longer* — or greater chance of living free of debilitating accidents, illnesses, diseases, and bodily malfunction.

_____

_____

_____

_____

_____

_____

_____

_____

_____

_____

_____

_____

_____

_____

_____

_____

_____

_____

_____

_____

_____

_____

_____

I thank you, God, for the opportunity to live my life this way.

........................., please do *everything you can* to assist me in creating lifelong healthy-weight living in a positive, pleasurable way. This benefits me *greatly*. I realize you're now doing it, and I thank you for it.

Living in my healthy-weight range is a *mandatory,* <u>must</u>-have feature of my existence. I am doing it *now* and for the rest of my life — and doing it *easily* <u>and</u> *enjoyably*. Yes! Yes! YES!

*   *   *

NOTE: After delivering the directive, close your eyes and say your Healthy-weight Goal Statement <u>three</u> times. Do it with intensity. ~ Plus, each day allow yourself to get a *good feeling* from making your weight losses stick and from having realized healthy-weight living. You deserve it. It's a substantial praiseworthy achievement.

> The **Weight Success Benefits Directive** is an important message for your mind, especially your subconscious mind. Deliver it like it is and your subconscious mind will act accordingly.

How to Deliver the Weight Success Benefits Directive for Maximal Effect

For extra impact, consider applying creative delivery techniques when reading the Weight Success Benefits Directive. Doing this can cause your mind — especially your subconscious mind — to pay extra attention to what you're telling it to do. Here are five examples to consider.

First, emphasize the key words. You can do this by speaking slightly louder, or slower, or more forcefully. These key words are printed in *italic,* underline, or **bold.**

Second, repeat (reread) a particular phrase or sentence for emphasis. So, what parts should you be focusing on? Reread whichever actions of the five directive actions you feel are most relevant at the time. If you happen to be in a period of progress slowdown, it likely means some action called for by the Directive is not being fully performed by your subconscious mind. So, emphasize to your mind that you definitely want it to be doing this action.

Third, read the entire Directive slowly and deliberately. This will require one or two extra minutes. But it can pay dividends. It can cause your subconscious mind to pay special attention to the instructions contained in the Directive. To do this, pause for a few seconds after each action or paragraph. During the pause, reflect on the meaning or main message of the action.

Fourth, ad lib whenever you see fit. Insert spontaneous additional instructions to your subconscious mind to emphasize key points or actions.

Fifth, deliver the Directive in a different place or position. For example, if you've been delivering the Directive sitting down, do it standing. Or, deliver it while pacing, like you're delivering a speech. Include arm movement and gesticulation of main points. This can be a powerful form of delivery. It can enhance your emotional impact. Experiment and find out what works best for you. Or, just change delivery style from time to time for variety.

Also, if there's a word in the directive and you'd like to delete it, just draw a line through it. If you'd like to replace it with a different word, write in the new word above the word that has the line through it.

> For more instructions on the Directive, go to the *Detailed Instructions for Weight Success Benefits Directive* chapter (p. **85**). Reading this is recommended.

Daily Action 4: GOAL STATEMENT
Each day, say your Healthy-weight Goal Statement at least 25 times.

This action typically takes <u>*less than*</u> 120 seconds.

To do it you need a healthy-weight goal statement. The one I recommend (and have been personally using since 2008) is this:

> *I <u>am</u> the person of my healthy weight.*
> *I am healthy, happy, and doing great.*

As previously explained, every weight in your healthy-weight range is considered to be a *healthy weight* for you.

WHY You Do It

Saying your Goal Statement each day focuses your mind — in particular, your subconscious mind — on the desired ultimate outcome of your healthy-weight pursuit. This triggers your subconscious mind to create daily thoughts and feelings that guide you toward right eating and living your life in your healthy-weight range.

HOW to Do It

Each day say your Healthy-weight Goal Statement at least 25 times. (Note: 25 times is a minimum, not a maximum. You can say it more than 25 times, if you like.) Does saying it 25 times a day seem like it would be time-consuming? It's not. You're able to say your Goal Statement *three times* in 12 to 15 seconds, which is 12 to 15 times a minute. Which means, saying it 25 times per day uses *less than* 120 seconds per day. So there's no reason why you can't do this Daily Action 4 every day.

Plus, the Goal Statement need not be said all at once. You can divide it into several sessions. Or, if you like, you can spread it throughout the day.

Plus, you can say it aloud, either in full voice or in a whisper. Or, you can say it silently to yourself — your choice. So, you can do this Action 4 *any time, any place*. Also, you can vary the *way* you say the statement from time to time. Sometimes do it more rapidly, other times more slowly. And, for variety put emphasis on different words at different times.

Plus, you can fit them into "free time." Each of your days contains numerous "free time" periods where statement iterations can be fit in. These periods are when you're doing something but also can be thinking about something else at the same time. Examples include when you're lying in bed, dressing, showering, driving, walking from here to there, taking a break, eating, using the bathroom, exercising, and watching TV. So, each day holds opportunities where you can fit in five or ten iterations of your Healthy-weight Goal Statement. Because you're doing this while also doing something else, you can consider the time involved to be non-dedicated time, or free time. In short, there are so many opportunities for free-time statement iteration you can, if you wish, easily fit 40, 50, or even 100 or more into a day without any special time allotment.

Plus, here's an easy way to keep tract of your goal statement iterations: Count them in units of five using one of your hands. After each iteration move one of your fingers (either in or out). After moving all five fingers, say the total number to that point. So, after counting the first five say "Five" (either aloud or silently), after the second five say "Ten," after the third five "Fifteen," and so on.

Even though you can say your Goal Statement any time you want, some particularly good times to say it are (a) when you awaken in the morning, (b) whenever you feel an urge to eat, (c) *while you're eating*, (d) before you go to sleep at night, and (e) whenever you wake up in the night. Saying it at these times can have extra-powerful impact.

Finally, whenever you're saying your Healthy-weight Goal Statement — either aloud or silently in your mind — *hold the belief* that your mind is right then in the process of transforming you into the person described in the Statement — that is, "the person of your healthy weight" and one that's "healthy, happy, and doing great." Also, *act as-if*, or totally pretend, you're that person. Believing and acting as-if motivate your mind — in particular, your subconscious mind — to create the types of thoughts and feelings that steer you toward lifelong healthy-weight living. For more on this, go to the *How Believing and Acting As-if Work* section in Startup Action 5 (p. **38**).

> Also, consider applying optional backup depiction statements. For this, go to the *Motivator 2* section (p. **110**) in the *Six More Mind Motivators* chapter.

SUMMING UP This Daily Action 4

Each day say your Healthy-weight Goal Statement at least **25** times. You can say it any way you like (including silently to yourself) and also any time you like. But always say it at least once before each eating session. ~ Do this Daily Action 4, and also the other four daily actions of the Weight Success Method, and lifelong healthy-weight living will be *yours*.

REMEMBER: The secret to succeeding at lifelong healthy-weight living is: Do Weight Success Actions <u>every</u> day. You accomplish this by doing the Weight Success Method, which typically takes <u>less than</u> **8** minutes of dedicated time per day. This causes vital *success drivers* to be included in your weight success pursuit.

Daily Action 5: GUIDED EATING

Each time you eat, apply the Guided Eating Process.

This action typically takes *less than* 15 to 20 seconds of <u>non</u>-dedicated time per meal.

In any given eating session we pursue eating in one of two modes: (1) unguided or (2) guided.

Unguided Eating. Eating activity that's not guided by the eater — meaning, it's done automatically and without conscious deliberation — we call *unguided eating*. So, with unguided eating we don't guide our eating actions. Instead, the food items around us do that. These food items are visual cues. The cues trigger a certain behavior. This certain behavior consists of performing a series of eating actions that results in consuming the cues. We mostly perform this behavior automatically, or with minimal deliberation or conscious direction. (Note: Other names for unguided eating are automatic eating, undirected eating, and non-controlled eating.)

So, unguided eating is a 3-action process. First, we confront food items, which are cues. Second, the food cues trigger an automatic-eating response. Third, we engage in undirected or automatic eating until the cues disappear from being eaten. During this time we aren't thinking about what we're doing. As a result, we're not guiding our eating activity. For most persons nearly all eating is unguided. This is why many folks engage in frequent overeating — and, thereby, fail at creating healthy-weight living. So we should replace unguided eating with guided eating.

> For more on unguided eating, go to the *Key to Beating the Bad Habit of Unguided Eating* chapter (p. **152**).

Guided Eating. In guided eating *we* guide the eating process. Meaning, instead of the food items determining what and how much we eat, *we* do it. This might sound hard to do, but it's not. You can easily create guided eating any time you want. To do this, apply a certain 3-action process which we call *Guided Eating Process*. (Other names for guided eating are directed eating and controlled

eating.) Guided eating is a *major* key to replacing overweight living with healthy-weight living for life.

> **Note:** In this book the word *eating* encompasses drinking. And the word *food* encompasses beverages. So wherever you read the terms *eating* and *food* know that it includes drinking and beverages.

WHY You Do It

Whenever you're not guiding your eating activity, your eating activity is <u>un</u>controlled. This is why unguided eating leads to overeating. Doing this Daily Action 5 *reduces* the amount of unguided eating and *increases* the amount of guided eating. Which makes for *non*-overeating meals. This, in turn, leads you to weight success.

HOW to Do It

To create guided eating in any particular meal or eating session, apply this guided eating process: **C**ommunicate, **B**elieve, **A**ppreciate. It's your key to easy guided eating.

> **TIP:** To easily recall the three steps of the Guided Eating Process (**C**ommunicate, **B**elieve, **A**ppreciate), think of *C-B-A*. Which is *A-B-C in reverse*.

The C-B-A Guided Eating Process

Each time you eat perform these three steps.

1. **<u>C</u>ommunicate.** When you begin eating, deliver *guided-eating self-talk* to your self.

2. **<u>B</u>elieve.** As you eat, *hold the belief* and also act as-if your subconscious mind is right then, at that very moment, in the process of performing the actions described in your guided-eating self-talk. Which means, be on the lookout for a stop-eating signal.

3. **<u>A</u>ppreciate.** When a stop-eating signal comes, *thank* your subconscious mind for sending the signal and then <u>act on it</u> — that is, *stop eating*.

Doing this process takes no extra time. It's done on non-dedicated time, or while you're eating. Here's fuller explanation of how to do the three C-B-A steps.

Step 1: COMMUNICATE

Whenever you start eating, deliver guided-eating self-talk to your self. *Guided-eating self-talk* is any message delivered to your self while eating, for the purpose of causing your subconscious mind to assist with guiding you away from overeating and toward non-overeating. You can deliver self-talk either by whispering to yourself or by speaking silently in your mind. Do it whichever way works best for you at the time. To deliver guided-eating self-talk, do these two actions:

1 – Say your Healthy-weight Goal Statement;

2 – Describe how you want the eating session to turn out.

I'll explain these two actions.

ACTION 1: Silently say your Healthy-weight Goal Statement <u>three</u> times when you start eating. This takes only about 15 seconds. The Statement is:

> I <u>am</u> the person of my healthy weight.
> I am healthy, happy, and doing great.

ACTION 2: Silently tell your subconscious mind how you want the upcoming eating session to turn out. For this, use one or both of the following two guided-eating statements, *or* something like them. Either way, the object is to describe how you want the eating session to be.

Sample Guided-eating Self-talk Statement #1

This food is filling me up, filling me up, <u>filling me up</u>. I might not be able to eat it all.

Sample Guided-eating Self-talk Statement #2

This food is very, very, <u>very</u> satisfying. By the time I finish eating it I'll be <u>fully</u> satisfied and have <u>no</u> desire to eat any more this meal.

Now, both these statements refer to whatever amount of food constitutes a right amount for that meal. Typically it's the food that's on your plate or in hand, not everything on the table or in the refrigerator. Or, it's the amount of food prescribed by your preferred dietary program.

Also, if you like you can combine the two self-talk statements, like this:

This food is filling me up, filling me up, <u>filling me up</u>. I might not be able to eat it all. It's also very, very, <u>very</u> satisfying. By the time I finish eating it I'll be <u>fully</u> satisfied and have <u>no</u> desire to eat any more this meal.

Doing this triggers your subconscious mind to cause you to feel both filled up and fully sated with eating pleasure without overeating.

Note: the above statements are given as samples. If you so choose you can deviate from them or add to them. In short, ad lib whenever you feel like it. Also, to reiterate, you deliver guided-eating self-talk either by whispering or by speaking silently in your mind.

> For more on communicating to your subconscious mind, go to the "Six Actions for an Effective Thank You, Keep It Up Message" (p. **47**).

Step 2: BELIEVE

As you eat, hold the belief and also act as-if your subconscious mind is right then, at the present moment, in the process of performing the actions described in your guided-eating self-talk. Which means, as you're eating be on the lookout for a stop-eating signal. That is, expect that your mind will be creating a stop-eating signal at the point you should cease eating. (Note: It likely will include the full-stomach feeling.) Coming up on page 58 is a list of possible stop-eating signals.

> For more on believing and acting as-if, go to the *How Believing and Acting As-if Work* section in Startup Action 5 (p. **38**).

Step 3: APPRECIATE

When a stop-eating signal comes, thank your subconscious mind for sending the signal and then <u>act on it</u> — that is, stop eating. How do you thank your subconscious mind? It's easy — like this:

"Subconscious mind, I thank you very much for sending the stop-eating signal. I really appreciate it."

And, how do you act on the signal? Immediately after getting just a slight full-stomach feeling, or any other form of stop-eating signal, stop eating. Do *not* eat "just a few more bites." Do *not* decide to "finish off" what's on your plate or in your hand. Instead, stop eating right then. And, if there's any leftover food, immediately discard it or push it out of reach or put it into the refrigerator for eating the next day.

It might seem like this would be hard to do. That's because most of us have, at one time or another, acquired an eat-it-all, fill-'er-up habit. But overcoming this habit is easier than you might imagine. To do so, immediately follow the stop-eating signal when it comes. When you do this the urge to continue eating *immediately begins to fade away*. Which means, within about 30 to 60 seconds after you stop eating you no longer have an urge to continue eating.

And don't forget, after the signal comes, express appreciation and thanks to your subconscious mind for sending it. Conveying this thanks motivates your mind to keep assisting by sending further stop-eating signals when needed. Note: You can convey thanks by speaking either aloud, such as in a whisper, or silently in your mind — your choice.

When you do this Step 3 you get a bonus. You get a great feeling from having turned a potential overeating situation into a non-overeating victory. And, believe me, this feeling is way more gratifying than any feeling you get from continuing to eat.

At this point you might be thinking, "What happens if one ignores the stop-eating signal?" When you fail to follow a stop-eating signal — that is, when you continue eating or proceed into overeating — your mind retracts the signal. As a result, the feeling or thought that constituted the signal fades away. And, in its place, the "old" urge and habit to pursue overeating usually reappears.

What's more, if you repeatedly ignore the stop-eating signals your subconscious mind sends, it will eventually stop sending stop-eating signals. They become weaker and weaker over time.

Some Common Stop-eating Signals

Here's a list of seven common signals your subconscious mind might use for telling you to stop eating or to refrain from eating.

1. The full-stomach feeling. This typically involves a feeling of pressure or tightening at the top of your stomach, or where your stomach joins your throat. Even just a slight full-stomach feeling is a stop-eating signal. This feeling can come even when your stomach isn't completely full. The full-stomach feeling is likely the most common, or #1, stop-eating signal.

2. A reduced urge to eat or to continue eating. Even just a slightly-reduced urge is a stop-eating signal.

3. The food you're eating or thinking of eating suddenly loses its appeal or begins to "lose its taste." Even just a slight reduction in the food's appeal or taste is a stop-eating signal.

4. A feeling or suspicion that if you eat a certain food or a certain amount of food it will give you a bloated or overly-full feeling. Even just a slight feeling that this might happen is a stop-eating, or don't-eat-it, signal.

5. A thought of something you haven't yet done but that needs doing.

6. A thought of something you need to say to someone.

7. An urge to pursue some other activity, with this other activity being a non-eating activity. Even just a slight urge to pursue another activity is a stop-eating signal.

A stop-eating or don't-eat-it signal typically involves one or both of two types of actions: deactivating and diverting. The first three actions in the above list are *deactivating* actions. The last four are *diverting* actions. Also, it's possible your subconscious mind might devise a stop-eating signal not on this list! So be on the alert for some new form of stop-eating signal your mind might devise.

How to Trigger a Stop-eating or Don't-eat-it Signal. The key to having your subconscious mind send a stop-eating signal before the point of overeating is this. Make sure you're applying Step 2 — the Believing or "B" step (p. **57**) — of the Guided Eating Process. This puts you on the lookout for the signal. Which, in turn, causes your subconscious mind to send it. But, if you like you can do more. Try this handy technique. Pause your eating for a few seconds and then whisper or silently say to yourself: *Subconscious mind, have I eaten enough? If so, send me the full-stomach feeling this very moment.*

Then focus on your stomach. If you sense just the slightest feeling of "change" or pressure or fullness in your stomach or where your stomach joins your throat, that's a stop-eating signal. So stop eating right then. When you do this — that is, follow the signal — the urge to continue eating *immediately begins to fade away.*

Conversely, if your subconscious mind doesn't send you a stop-eating signal when you ask "Have I eaten enough?" it could mean that you haven't overeaten at that time. Or, if you complete a meal and never get a stop-eating signal it might mean that your subconscious mind has concluded that eating that amount of food at that time will lead you to having an overeating-free day.

During-eating Self-talk — *Powerful!*

Now and then you might find yourself in a situation that appears like it could lead to overeating — like, for example, a super-strong eating urge or an extra-tempting meal. For this you can apply extra guided-eating self-talk. We call it *during-eating self-talk.* Here's how to do it.

First, make sure you do the self-talk prescribed for Step 1 of the Guided Eating Process (p. **56**). *Then, include additional self-talk as you're eating.* Every couple minutes or so, silently describe to yourself the way that eating session is, or should be, turning out. If you like, you can silently repeat the initial two Guided-eating Self-talk Statements (p. **57**). Every time you deliver this self-talk, hold the belief and act as-if your subconscious mind is right then in the process of bringing about the situation depicted in the self-talk message. For more on believing and acting as-if, go to the *How Believing and Acting As-if Work* section in Startup Action 5 (p. **38**).

This tactic might seem gimmicky, but it's powerful. During-eating self-talk is your never-fail SWAT team for neutralizing mealtime overeating and turning any eating session into an overeating-

free victory. Use it anytime you need to stifle over-eating.

Snack-time Procrastination

The prior-described during-eating self-talk tactic works for defeating overeating during extra-tempting meals. But now and then you might have need to defeat overeating that arises from eating too much between meals, called over-snacking.

When you're grappling with over-snacking you might apply the *procrastinate tactic.* That is, don't decide to not snack; instead just postpone the decision. Tell yourself you'll take up the matter in a little while, perhaps *after* completing some activity. In doing this you avoid the snacking self-argument. You don't become involved with the question "Should I snack, or should I not?" So, you don't end up enflaming the snacking urge by making a don't-snack decision. Instead, you sidestep it by postponing the decision. When you do this the snacking urge dissipates as soon as you start pursuing the other activity. Usually that's the only time you'll need to deal with the snacking urge for that portion of the day. But, what do you do if some time later the snacking urge reappears? You do what all good procrastinators do: You procrastinate again.

SUMMING UP This Daily Action 5

Each time you eat do guided eating with the C-B-A process: **(1) C**OMMUNICATE guided-eating self-talk to your self — including to your subconscious mind, **(2) B**ELIEVE and act as-if your mind is in the process of doing what you're describing, and when a stop-eating signal comes, **(3) A**PPRECIATE the signal, thank your subconscious mind for it, and *immediately stop eating.* When you do this the urge to continue eating immediately begins to fade away. ~ Do this Daily Action 5, plus the other four Daily Actions, and lifelong healthy-weight living will be *yours.*

For deeper insight into *why* the Weight Success Method works, read the *Why the Weight Success Method Gets Your Whole Mind Involved* chapter (p. **129**) and the *How the Weight Success Method Enhances Your Life Journey* chapter (p. **157**).

(i) Essence of Chapter Two and This Book

AT THIS POINT we provide a distillation of the core concepts of this Chapter Two — which also are the core concepts of this book.

The ultimate purpose of the pursuit of weight management is to create weight success. Formally defined, *weight success* is: Living most or all of one's days in one's desired healthy-weight range <u>and</u> deriving benefits, enjoyment, and fulfillment from it. So, there are two parts to weight success: (1) creating the situation of living in one's desired healthy-weight range — otherwise called *healthy-weight living* — and (2) realizing benefits, enjoyment, and fulfillment from it.

There's a certain core activity required for creating lifelong healthy-weight living. It's this:

Do Weight Success Actions every day.

We call this the **Weight Success Secret.**

Formally defined, a *Weight Success Action* is an action that contributes to creating weight success. By doing Weight Success Actions every day we create Weight Success Days. This book presents a plethora of examples of Weight Success Actions, which includes: the ten Startup Actions (p. 35), the five Daily Actions (p. 44), and nearly all the actions described in Part B (p. 70–182).

To enable you to easily do the most vital Weight Success Actions every day this book provides a powerful weight success methodology. Formally defined, a *weight success methodology* is an action plan that consists of specific weight success actions that, when performed by a person, causes a maximal number of success drivers to be included in a weight success pursuit, thereby resulting in easiest possible creation of weight success. We've dubbed the weight success methodology presented in this book **Weight Success Method.**

Doing the Weight Success Method results in most or all of nineteen powerful success drivers being included in your weight success pursuit. Formally defined, a *success driver* is a condition or activity that, when present, increases the likelihood of you succeeding at a certain pursuit.

In essence, the Weight Success Method is a special set of ten Startup Actions done at the beginning of your weight success pursuit, followed by five Daily Actions done every day of the pursuit. The five Daily Actions consist of (1) Weighing, (2) Reinforcement or Correction, (3) Benefits Directive, (4) Goal Statement, and (5) Guided Eating. Doing all five typically takes <u>less than</u> **8** minutes of dedicated time per day.

Within all this there operates a certain core dynamic. We dub it *Weight Success Dynamic*. It's this: Doing the Weight Success Method each day installs success drivers into one's weight success pursuit which, in turn, results in experiencing weight success. It's depicted by the following infographic:

WEIGHT SUCCESS DYNAMIC

| Doing Weight Success METHOD each day | installs | Success DRIVERS into Weight Pursuit | which creates | Experiencing Weight SUCCESS |

WEIGHT SUCCESS = Living most or all of one's days in one's desired healthy-weight range <u>and</u> deriving benefits, enjoyment, and fulfillment from it. ~ For description of benefits created by weight success, see Chapter 7 (p. **80**). For description of enjoyment and fulfillment created by doing the Weight Success Method and achieving healthy-weight living, go to Chapter 17 (p. **123**), Chapter 22 (p. **157**), and Chapter 24 (p. **168**). ~ A person who's in process of creating weight success we call a *Weight Winner.*

(j) Lifelong Weight Success Empowerment

How the Weight Success Dynamic enables the skill of lifelong weight success empowerment.

YOU'VE LEARNED of the Weight Success Dynamic in prior discussion. We've depicted it in infographic form, including on prior page 60. It's a dynamic that consists of three factors connected by two impact bridges, one of the bridges being indicated by the word "installs" and the other by "which creates."

But it also can be expressed in text, like this. *Doing the Weight Success Method each day installs success drivers into one's weight success pursuit which, in turn, results in experiencing weight success.*

As previously stated, we define weight success as: Living most or all of one's days in one's desired healthy-weight range <u>and</u> deriving benefits, enjoyment, and fulfillment from it.

Now, a question arises: How long will the Weight Success Dynamic <u>continue</u>? This is a vital question, because for every 10 persons who lose weight about 9 of them are gaining it back, or going from "weight success" to "weight failure."

The answer to that question is this: The Weight Success Dynamic can continue *for the rest of your life* ... and will do so with just a reasonable amount of diligence by you.

Why does this happen? It's because there's a <u>third</u> impact bridge in the Weight Success Dynamic (depicted by the blue line in the infographic below). It extends from the Success block to the Method block and includes the words "which promotes continuation of." This bridge exists because of *positive reinforcement*. It works like this.

Upon achieving weight success via doing the Weight Success Method a person comes into a wonderful situation. They're now living all or most of their days in their desired healthy-weight range <u>and</u> deriving benefits, enjoyment, and fulfillment from it.

> The text under the infographic on the prior page tells where to go to get a description of these benefits.

The "benefits, enjoyment, and fulfillment" part of weight success is *positive reinforcement* that promotes continuation of doing the Weight Success Method.

Summed up, weight success acts as positive reinforcement that motivates continuation of doing the Weight Success Method or, put another way, weight success increases the likelihood of a person continuing to do the Method each day. This "continuation-promoting effect" of positive reinforcement works to propel the Weight Success Dynamic for life. So, we now relabel the Dynamic to include the word *Lifelong* in the name, as shown below.

Now here's the vital final point: This dynamic enables a person to develop an ability, or power, to create weight success for life. We call this ability ***Weight Success Empowerment.*** (It's depicted by the green portion in the infographic below.) Now this is what you need to know: I believe virtually anyone can acquire weight success empowerment by continually doing the Weight Success Method.

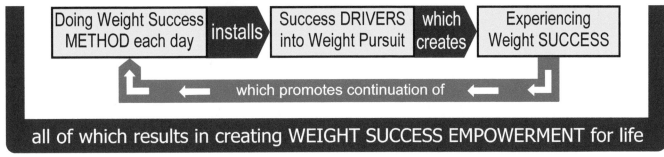

LIFELONG WEIGHT SUCCESS DYNAMIC

| Doing Weight Success METHOD each day | installs | Success DRIVERS into Weight Pursuit | which creates | Experiencing Weight SUCCESS |

which promotes continuation of

all of which results in creating WEIGHT SUCCESS EMPOWERMENT for life

(k) Why We've Been Struggling with Weight Control

Weight control — a.k.a. weight management — is the act of regulating one's amount of body fat for maintaining one's weight in a certain weight range.

TO WRAP UP this Chapter 2, I propose and then answer one of the most vexing questions of our time: Why have we, as a society, been struggling with weight control? To answer this question I present five key concepts. Three have already been introduced in this chapter and two are new. These concepts enable us to understand why achieving weight control has been such a widespread struggle in our modern world. Here they are.

1 – Primary Purpose of Eating

2 – Cause of Fat Gain

3 – Factors that Promote Overperformance of the O-I-S Process and Fat Gain

4 – New-situation Creation

5 – To Achieve Weight <u>Control</u>, Pursue Weight <u>Success</u>

We'll now examine each concept.

KEY CONCEPT 1:
Primary Purpose of Eating

Eating is a pleasurable experience. As such, humankind — or at least modern humankind — has come to assume that the primary purpose of eating is to derive maximal eating pleasure.

But this assumption is dangerous and destructive. How so? It's because when we assume that the primary purpose of eating is to derive maximal eating pleasure it causes an undesired outcome; it causes us to engage in overeating, which results in continual weight gain, which results in continual overweight living.

So, what is, or should be, the primary purpose of eating? The primary purpose of eating should be: To consume the *types* of food and the *amount* of food that contributes to (a) creating optimal health and (b) living in one's healthy-weight range.

Once we are accomplishing the primary purpose of eating on a daily basis, then we add in a secondary purpose of eating: Deriving eating pleasure in conjunction with accomplishing the primary purpose. For easy reference we call this right eating. So, *right eating* is: Eating right foods in right amounts and in a way that creates right eating enjoyment. Right eating is the roadway to lifelong healthy-weight living.

> More information on this subject can be found in "Startup Action 6: Eating Approach," page 39.

KEY CONCEPT 2:
Cause of Fat Gain

One of the biggest impediments to weight control in modern society is that we've become confused over what is the *cause* of fat gain. So here's the nitty-gritty on it (previously explained in Startup Action 1, page 35).

Fat gain is caused by one — and only one — thing: overeating. We define *overeating* as: Consuming more calories than what one's body is metabolizing, or "burning up," per day.

Or, put another way, the cause of fat gain is *overperformance* of a certain three-action process, the process of:

1 – Opening our mouth;

2 – Inserting a piece of metabolizable calorie-containing food into our mouth; and

3 – Swallowing the piece of food.

We call it the *Open–Insert–Swallow* process — or **O-I-S** process for short. Overperformance, or over-repetition, of this process is the <u>real</u> cause of overeating and weight gain. And, it's the only cause. This process is how we consume more metabolizable calories than what our body is metabolizing, or "burning up," per day, which in turn causes us to gain fat and to struggle with achieving weight control. And, finally, it's important to note that this O–I–S process is totally controllable by each of us.

So, what about all the "zillion" other factors that researchers and writers of the past thirty years have been "discovering" and calling the "cause" of weight gain and overweight living?

KEY CONCEPT 3:
Factors that Promote Overperformance of the O-I-S Process and Fat Gain

Even though there is only one cause of fat gain, which is overeating — a.k.a. overperformance of the Open–Insert–Swallow process — there's a slew of factors that promote fat gain. Or, put another way, there are dozens, maybe hundreds, of factors that promote or facilitate doing overeating and deriving fat gain from it. For simplicity I call these factors fat-promoting factors. I define *fat-promoting factors* as: Factors that promote overeating or fat gain, or make it easier for a person to overeat and gain weight.

> A list of fat-promoting factors can be found in a "Fat-promoting Factors" discussion on page 20.

But, in my opinion, of all the many fat-promoting factors five of them stand out as being most powerful in promoting overeating and in making us struggle with weight control. They are:

1 – Hunger pangs;

2 – Eating pleasure;

3 – Non-satiability of eating pleasure;

4 – Endless opportunity to experience instant eating pleasure; and

5 – Habit of unguided eating.

I refer to them as the "Big Five" of fat-promoting factors. I also call them Weight-control Inhibiting Factors, a term I'll be using in this discussion.

Weight-control Inhibiting Factor 1:
Hunger Pangs

The first major factor that has been promoting overeating and inhibiting our efforts to achieve weight control is that when we're involved in undereating we experience hunger, or hunger pangs. This experience is distinctly annoying or even painful, so we strive to avoid it. But undereating is necessary for weight reduction. And, brief periods of temporary weight reduction are necessary for most people to achieve ongoing weight control — a.k.a. lifelong healthy-weight living. So, refusal to experience any form of hunger pang, even briefly, has been deterring our achievement of weight control.

Why do we experience hunger pangs? Most likely it's a feature of our human species that has arisen through evolutionary process. By motivating us to obtain and consume food to nullify the hunger pang, this feature results in us acquiring the physical sustenance we need to survive and reproduce, which results in continuation of our species.

Weight-control Inhibiting Factor 2:
Eating Pleasure

The second major factor that has been promoting overeating and inhibiting our efforts to achieve weight control is that eating is a distinctly pleasurable experience for us. Most people enjoy this pleasure a lot. But when the desire to experience this pleasure becomes priority #1 it triggers overeating. And, this has been deterring our achievement of weight control.

Why do we experience eating pleasure? Again, most likely it's a feature of our species that has arisen through evolutionary process. By us deriving pleasure from eating, it motivates us to create eating occasions, which results in us acquiring the physical sustenance we need to survive and reproduce.

So, the act of eating produces two simultaneous desired results. First, it causes an immediate reduction in pain (by removing any hunger pang) and, second, it provides an immediate jolt of pleasure (in the form of eating pleasure). As such, hunger pangs and eating pleasure are flipsides of a same "eating stimulus coin." Together, they work as an evolutionarily created double-whammy that moves us to constantly seek out or create eating occasions.

Weight-control Inhibiting Factor 3:
Non-satiability of Eating Pleasure

The third major factor that has been promoting overeating and inhibiting our efforts to achieve weight control is that we seldom tire of experiencing eating pleasure.

Many types of pleasures can become boring to us, or somehow decline in strength, or diminish in appeal. But not so with food. Eating pleasure seems to be non-satiable. We seem to never tire of it or lose interest in experiencing it every day. Indeed, it seems to work "in reverse," the more we experience of it, the more we seem to want it. This non-satiability of eating pleasure triggers overeating, which has been deterring our achievement of weight control.

Why does this situation exist? Again, perhaps it's an evolutionarily created feature of our species that serves to perpetuate the species. Or, perhaps it's an evolutionarily created feature "run amok."

Weight-control Inhibiting Factor 4:
Endless Opportunity to Experience Instant Eating Pleasure

The fourth major factor that has been promoting overeating and inhibiting our efforts to achieve weight control is that in modern society there is endless opportunity to experience instant eating pleasure. Meaning, it's because readily consumable food is everywhere. So most persons, or those not living in severe poverty, have the easy opportunity to eat any time, any place.

Having universal abundance of instantly consumable food is a huge blessing, but it also can be a trap. In prior centuries eating required special preparation and work. So eating was confined to a few (such as three) distinct eating sessions per day. And, each eating session had boundaries, a beginning and an ending.

But with readily consumable food everywhere, the natural boundaries of eating have tended to fade away. No longer is work required for eating and no longer are there beginning and ending points. Instead, eating has morphed into an effortless process that tends to flow through every day without major interruption or lengthy breaks. As a result, this situation of having universal abundance of instantly consumable food promotes overeating, which has been deterring our achievement of weight control.

Each of weight-control inhibiting factors 1, 2, and 3 is, in itself, a powerful force for promoting overeating and weight gain and, thereby, it's a powerful factor deterring weight control. But, when factors 1–3 are joined by this factor 4, overeating and weight gain become supercharged, and weight control becomes a daunting challenge. This is the predicament that modern society is in today.

Weight-control Inhibiting Factor 5:
Habit of Unguided Eating

The fifth major factor that has been promoting overeating and inhibiting our efforts to achieve weight control is that the activity of unguided eating has become a deeply ingrained habit with most humans. This habit results in overeating, and this, in turn, has been deterring our achievement of weight control.

> **Definition for review:** *Unguided eating* is eating that's not guided by the eater; it's eating that's done automatically and without conscious deliberation.

Why do we have this habit? It's because the activity of unguided eating is an activity that starts shortly after birth and is then repeated numerous times every day thereafter, resulting in *thousands* of repetitions every year. This constant daily repetition of unguided eating makes it become a strong, deeply ingrained habit that promotes daily overeating.

> For more on unguided eating, see "Daily Action 5: Guided Eating" (p. 56). ~ For more on habits, see the *Key to Beating the Bad Habit of Unguided Eating* chapter (p. 152).

Summation of the "Big Five" Weight-control Inhibiting Factors

We now provide a summary.

Weight control is the act of regulating one's amount of body fat for maintaining one's weight in a certain desired weight range. Many factors — a.k.a. fat-promoting factors — can affect the degree of difficulty in achieving weight control. But, in my opinion, five factors have been having an outsized impact on inhibiting the achievement of weight control within modern society. I call them the "Big Five" Weight-control Inhibiting Factors, or WCIF for short. In summary, they work like this.

WCIF #1: *Hunger Pangs.* This factor deters weight reduction by making undereating to be a pain-producing experience.

WCIF #2: *Eating Pleasure.* This factor promotes weight gain by making eating, including overeating, to be a pleasure-producing experience.

WCIF #3: *Non-satiability of Eating Pleasure.* This factor promotes weight gain by making eating, including overeating, to be a pleasure-producing experience we never tire of.

WCIF #4: *Endless Opportunity to Experience Instant Eating Pleasure.* This factor promotes weight gain by making eating, including overeating, to be an easy, instantaneous pleasure-producing experience that can be had any time of every day.

WCIF #5: *Habit of Unguided Eating.* This factor promotes weight gain by making eating, including overeating, to be a habitual unguided activity that happens automatically, or without deliberate conscious thought, every day.

> **Definitions for review:** *Under-eating* is consuming fewer calories than what your body is metabolizing, or "burning up," per day. ~ *Overeating* is consuming more calories than what your body is metabolizing, or "burning up," per day.

This brings us to the fourth key concept.

> ## KEY CONCEPT 4:
> ### New-situation Creation

"Life-enhancing situation" is a key term in this discussion. I define *life-enhancing situation* as: a new situation that's an improvement over a present situation. The story of humankind is a story of an endless pursuit of creating life-enhancing situations.

There are two main ways we create life-enhancing situations. The first way is we eradicate a particular factor that's causing a problem at the present time. I call this *causal-factor eradication.* The second way is we create a desired *new* situation that, when actualized, automatically replaces a non-desired present situation. I call this *new-situation creation.* Here's how these two approaches work.

Causal-factor Eradication

Causal-factor eradication involves four actions.

First, we identify a problem or malady we'd like to eliminate.

Second, we identify the cause of the malady — a.k.a. causal factor.

Third, we identify, obtain, or create an antidote that, when applied, will eradicate the causal factor.

Fourth, we apply the antidote and, thereby, eliminate or nullify the causal factor, which results in eliminating the problem or malady.

Causal-factor eradication can be best illustrated using the field of medicine. This approach is how we free our self from a medical problem. First, we identify a particular sickness, illness, ailment, or malady we'd like to be free of. Second, we identify the causal factor that's creating the malady. Third, we obtain or create an antidote that, when applied, will eradicate the causal factor. Fourth, we apply the antidote, which results in curing or mitigating the sickness, thereby creating a life-enhancing situation. The antidote typically involves some sort of injection, pill, medication, surgery, or activity that reduces, eliminates, or overrides the illness-causing factor.

New-situation Creation

The second main way we create life enhancement is we create a desired *new* situation that, when actualized, automatically replaces a non-desired present situation. For this to work, the desired new situation and the non-desired present situation must be mutually exclusive. That is, only one of the situations can exist at a time. For example, right eating and overeating are mutually exclusive situations;

the presence of one rules out, or nullifies, the presence of the other.

The new-situation creation approach to creating a life-enhancing situation involves four actions.

First, we identify, describe, and envision the desired new situation we want to create or have actualized.

Second, we identify the factors required for succeeding at creating the desired new situation. We call these factors success-creation drivers, or success drivers for short.

> **Definition for review:** A *success driver* is a condition or activity that, when present, increases the likelihood of a person succeeding at a certain pursuit — or, more specifically, increases the likelihood of a person performing actions that contribute to creating a certain desired situation or outcome associated with the pursuit. ~ (More information on success drivers can be found on page 23.)

Third, we obtain or formulate a methodology — a.k.a. success methodology — that, when enacted, will bring success drivers into the pursuit of creating the desired new situation.

> **Definition for review:** A *success methodology* is an action plan that pertains to a certain pursuit and consists of specific actions that, when performed by a person, causes a maximal number of success drivers to be included in that pursuit, thereby resulting in easiest possible creation of the desired situation or outcome associated with the pursuit. ~ (More information on success methodology can be found on page 22.)

Fourth, we do the success methodology — that is, we perform the actions described in the action plan. By doing this we actualize the desired new situation. And, because the desired new situation and the non-desired present situation are mutually exclusive, the desired new situation replaces the non-desired present situation, thereby resulting in life enhancement.

Although most people haven't realized it, the above two approaches to creating life enhancement — the causal-factor eradication approach and the new-situation creation approach — have been used for years, and each has played a key role in humankind's quest and creation of ongoing life enhancement. But, the results achieved from these two approaches can vary depending on the situation.

What's the Best Approach for Weight Control Success?

Some life-enhancing situations are most easily achieved via applying the causal-factor eradication approach. Other situations are most easily achieved via the new-situation creation approach. Now here is a sixth Weight-control Inhibiting Factor (in addition to the five previously described). As a society, we've been focusing on the least-effective approach to creating weight control. We've been trying to achieve weight control via application of the causal-factor eradication approach to creating life enhancement. But this endeavor has been less-than-fully effective. Indeed, it has been a dismal failure.

Why has that been the case? It's because the primary causal factor that's been creating the problem of fat gain and overweight living is not a condition or a thing. Rather, it's a *human activity* — specifically, it's the activity of daily overperforming the three-action process of opening our mouth, inserting food into our mouth, and swallowing the food. Now here's the rub. When human activity is a causal factor of a particular problem, that causal factor can be especially hard to eradicate. The reason for this is, in order for us humans to eradicate this causal factor we first must acknowledge that *we* — that is, our *controllable actions* — are the *cause* of the problem.

But, individually and as a society, we resist doing that. We do so because acknowledging that we — or our controllable actions — are the *cause* of the weight-gain problem is distressing and embarrassing to us. So, for the past 20 or so years, instead of acknowledging and addressing the *causal* factor of fat gain and overweight living — which is overeating, or consuming more calories than what our body is metabolizing per day — we've been diverting our attention to discovering and identifying sideline fat-promoting factors not related to our controllable actions but which promote overeating and fat gain. Then we've been acting as-if these sideline fat-promoting factors are "the cause" of our weight gain and weight control failure.

> **Definition for review.** A *fat-promoting factor* is a factor that promotes overeating or fat gain, or makes it easier for a person to overeat and gain weight (but isn't the cause of overeating or fat gain). As previously noted, there's a long list of fat-promoting factors provided on page 20, and also the five biggest of them are described in the "Summation of Big Five Weight-control Inhibiting Factors" section (p. 64).

So, the end-result is we've identified "zillions" of fat-promoting factors, and not one is the actual cause of fat gain and overweight living. These factors have become strawmen that we've set up as "the cause" of fat gain and weight control failure. This, in turn, enables us to cast the blame for our weight control failure onto these strawmen and, thereby, save face. But in spite of discovering a plethora of fat-promoting factors, we still haven't solved the overweightness problem. Indeed, the problem has actually grown. So, we remain in the undesired situation of not achieving weight control success. Which brings us to the question "What should we be doing now?"

One of the keys to achieving weight control success is: *Apply the new-situation creation approach to life enhancement.* As pertains to weight control, this process involves doing these four actions.

Action One: *Identify, describe, and envision the new situation that we desire to create, or to actualize.* As pertains to the pursuit of weight control, the desired new situation we seek to realize is lifelong healthy-weight living.

> **Definition review.** *Healthy-weight living* is: Living most or all of one's days in one's desired healthy-weight range.

Action Two: *Identify the factors required for succeeding at creating the desired new situation of lifelong healthy-weight living.* We've identified nineteen of these factors in this chapter (starting on page 23). For easy reference we call these factors success drivers.

> **Definition review.** A *success driver* is a condition or activity that, when present, increases the likelihood of a person succeeding at a certain pursuit — or, more specifically, increases the likelihood of a person perform-

ing actions that contribute to creating a certain desired situation or outcome associated with the pursuit.

Action Three: *Obtain or formulate a methodology — a.k.a. success methodology — that, when enacted, brings success drivers into our pursuit of creating the desired new situation of lifelong healthy-weight living.*

> **Definition review.** A *success methodology* is an action plan that pertains to a certain pursuit and consists of specific actions that, when performed by a person, causes a maximal number of success drivers to be included in that pursuit, thereby resulting in easiest possible creation of the desired situation or outcome associated with the pursuit.

As pertains to the pursuit of weight control, the most effective methodology we know is the *Weight Success Method,* described in this chapter starting on page 35.

Action Four: *Do the actions specified in the success methodology.* Which means, as pertains to the pursuit of weight control we do the actions described in the Weight Success Method. This method comprises two sets of actions: (a) startup actions and (b) daily actions. By doing these actions we actualize, or bring about, the desired new situation of lifelong healthy-weight living. And, because healthy-weight living and non-healthy-weight living — a.k.a. overweight living — are mutually exclusive, the desired new situation of healthy-weight living automatically replaces the "old" non-desired situation of non-healthy-weight living. Further, by continuing to do the daily actions specified in the Weight Success Method for the rest of our life we continue living in our healthy-weight range the rest of our life.

This Action Four of the weight control process can be distilled to an essence that's expressed in a single sentence, which is this: To succeed at lifelong healthy-weight living, do Weight Success Actions <u>every day</u>. For easy reference we've dubbed this activity *Weight Success Secret* (and described it on page 21).

> **Definition review.** A *Weight Success Action* is an action that contributes to creating weight success. Or, more specifically, it's an action that promotes living most or all of one's days in one's desired healthy-weight range <u>and</u> deriving benefits, enjoyment, and fulfillment from it.

Examples of Weight Success Actions include the ten Startup Actions, the five Daily Actions, the actions described in the Weight Success Benefits Directive, and any of the actions prescribed in section B of this book.

KEY CONCEPT 5:
To Achieve Weight Control, Pursue Weight Success

We begin this section with our initial definition. *Weight control* is the act of regulating one's amount of body fat for maintaining one's weight in a certain weight range. Individually and as a society, we've been struggling mightily to achieve weight control. But as a society we've been failing at it.

Now the time has come to disclose a little secret. The easiest, most effective way to achieve weight control is to aim *beyond* weight control. That is, strive to achieve *more* than weight control; strive to achieve weight *success*.

As defined throughout this Chapter 2, *weight success* is: Living most or all of one's days in one's desired healthy-weight range and deriving benefits, enjoyment, and fulfillment from it. When one is pursuing weight *success*, achieving weight *control* happens automatically. That's because weight control is no longer merely a "daily grinding must-do struggle." Instead, it becomes an exciting progress action, or uplifting daily step, in a greater quest, the quest of succeeding at creating lifelong healthy-weight living and deriving daily benefits, enjoyment, and fulfillment from it.

So, how does one put oneself on the road to lifelong weight success? You already know the answer: Do the success methodology known as *Weight Success Method*. Doing the Weight Success Method automatically activates a certain cause-effect chain that we call Lifelong Weight Success Dynamic (depicted on page 61). And, once this dynamic is operating a person acquires the ability or power to create personal weight success. We call this power *weight success empowerment*. A main purpose of this book is to enable and inspire you to acquire the ability of weight success empowerment, thereby enabling you to live most or all of the rest of your days in your desired healthy-weight range and derive benefits, enjoyment, and fulfillment from it.

For description of weight success benefits created by weight success, see Chapter 7 (p. **80**). For description of enjoyment and fulfillment created by doing the Weight Success Method and achieving weight success, go to Chapter 17 (p. **123**), Chapter 22 (p. **157**), and Chapter 24 (p. **168**).

What It's Fundamentally About

Some people think weight control success is an "Exercise Thing." Others think it's a "Dietary Thing." Still others think it's a "Medical Procedures Thing." But, fundamentally, it's a "MIND Thing." It's about creating thoughts and feelings that guide you to doing Weight Success Actions <u>every day</u>. That, in essence, is how lifelong weight control and weight success come about. The Weight Success Method is the easiest, most effective tool there is for making that happen.

~ **This concludes Chapter 2.** ~

We now sum up the essence of this chapter in a single sentence — which also sums up the essence of this book.

> To succeed at lifelong healthy-weight living,
> **do Weight Success Actions *every day*.**

By doing a certain amount of Weight Success Actions every day it causes you to *succeed* at creating lifelong healthy-weight living. (And, conversely, by <u>not</u> doing Weight Success Actions every day it likely results in you failing at creating healthy-weight living.)

The most powerful Weight Success Actions we know are the actions of the Weight Success Method. So, first do the ten *Startup* Actions (p. 35). Then, for the rest of your life do the five *Daily* Actions (p. 44) **every day.** (It typically takes *less than* eight minutes of dedicated time per day.)

The next most powerful Weight Success Actions we know are certain optional actions described in various chapters contained in Section B of this book. The chapters that contain specific optional actions include chapters 6–16, 21, and 27.

> Doing
> **Weight Success Actions**
> every day is the Way to
> **Lifelong Weight Success**

SECTION B:
OPTIONAL BACKUP RESOURCES

THIS SECTION is a powerful in-depth resource that provides additional information and insights for readers seeking extra knowledge or an answer to an outlying question. It comprises the following chapter titles (3 through 27).

CHAPTER 3: Model Day with the Weight Success Method

The Weight Success Method might look complex, but actually it's *simple and easy.* And, it typically takes *less than* 8 minutes of dedicated time per day.

TO ENSURE clarity I'm now going to provide an example: a fictional day that involves the five daily actions. This model day is presented in first-person singular, or as if it were happening to <u>me</u>. We'll assume I'm in weight maintenance mode, which I have been for a number of years now.

In this model day the first thing I do when I wake up in the morning is say my Healthy-weight Goal Statement three times. Shortly after that I weigh myself, in the buff. I apply the Eight Rules for Correct Daily Weighing (p. **45**). This is Daily Action 1. It takes only about 20 seconds.

When my daily weight reading is a desired reading, which it almost always is, I immediately deliver positive reinforcement to my subconscious mind. This includes the Thank You, Keep It Up message (p. **46**). While delivering this self-reinforcement, and afterward as well, I'm *holding the belief* and *acting as-if* my subconscious mind is right then listening to what I'm saying and is in the process of performing the actions described in the message. This is Daily Action 2A. It takes only about 30 to 40 seconds.

But if my daily weight reading happens to be an undesired reading, I skip Action 2A and do Action 2B instead. For this action I take immediate corrective action. For the next 24 to 48 hours I do under-eating, or consume far less calories than what I'm expending. This typically corrects the undesired situation in 24 hours. Doing this requires no extra dedicated time to do.

So, the weight reading I get in Daily Action 1 determines the following action that I do. When I get a desired reading I do Action 2A and not Action 2B. When I get an undesired reading I do Action 2B and not Action 2A. (For clarity, I note that I very seldom need to do Action 2B any more — maybe once or twice a year, if that.)

Shortly after completing Daily Actions 1 and 2A, I deliver the Weight Success Benefits Directive (p. **52**) to my mind. The Directive instructs my subconscious mind to perform certain actions that assist me with realizing right eating and healthy-weight living. Throughout the day I'm holding the belief and acting as-if it's performing these actions. This is Daily Action 3. It takes only about two to three minutes to do.

Also throughout the day I say my Healthy-weight Goal Statement at least 25 times. Often I end up saying it more than that. Some of the times I say it speaking aloud, and sometimes in a whisper, and some of the times I say it speaking silently, or in my mind. I often say it during the "free time" periods in my day, or when I'm doing something else at the same time. So I'm using non-dedicated time. When I say it I'm holding the belief and acting as-if my mind — in particular, my subconscious mind — is right then in the process of creating the types of thoughts and feelings that steer me toward being the person described in the Goal Statement. This is Daily Action 4. It takes less than 120 seconds of <u>non</u>-dedicated time per day.

When I eat I usually apply the 3-step Guided Eating Process — **C**ommunicating, **B**elieving, **A**ppreciating (p. **56**), called C-B-A for short. This helps me turn the session into guided eating, which steers me away from overeating. Also, I'm diligent about applying the Process during the last meal of the day, which usually is supper. I do this because the last meal is often the *make-it-or-break-it time;* it determines whether the day turns out to be a non-overeating day or an overeating day. This is Daily Action 5. It takes only about 15 to 20 seconds of <u>non</u>-dedicated time per meal to do.

After I go to bed at night I silently say my Healthy-weight Goal Statement at least three times before falling asleep. If I wake up in the night, such as for going to the bathroom, I silently say it at least three times as I'm going back to sleep.

CONCLUDING NOTE: The total time consumed by all five daily actions is *less than* eight minutes of dedicated time for the 24-hour day. To me, this is a miniscule investment for gaining years of non-overweight living and the weight success benefits that come with it.

Five Big Points

Enact these five powerful tips.

1 – Never stop. ❧ After achieving your desired weight or going into maintenance mode, do not do what many dieters do. Do not decide to "take a break" or to "coast for a while." If you take a break you'll likely gain back all the weight you lost. Instead, continue doing the Weight Success Method for life. Remember, it typically takes less than eight minutes of dedicated time per day.

2 – Routinize and habituate. ❧ Make doing the five Daily Actions a *routine* in your life. As much as possible, do each of the Actions the same time and place every day. In short, make doing them a *habit*.

3 – Feel good about it. ❧ Each day allow yourself to get a *good feeling* from living yet another day in your healthy-weight range. You deserve it. It's a substantial praiseworthy accomplishment.

4 – It has worked for the author for *over* ten years — it'll work for you, too. ❧ The writer of this book has been using and refining the Weight Success Method since 2007. He's been doing it because it works, and works easily. With it, you too can maintain your weight in your healthy-weight range the rest of your life *and* you can do it easily.

5 – Pursue it for what it is: a success-creation process. ❧ Remember this. To succeed at lifelong healthy-weight living, do Weight Success Actions every day. Any action that contributes to creating weight success qualifies as a Weight Success Action. Five very powerful Weight Success Actions are the five Daily Actions of the Weight Success Method. Doing these five actions typically takes *less than* **8** minutes of dedicated time per day. The result is it causes success drivers to be included in your weight success pursuit — which, in turn, results in you realizing lifelong weight success.

So, What's the Next Step?

Your next step in weight management decision-making could be one of the most impacting decisions of your life. If you make the decision to do nothing it'll likely result in ongoing weight gain and yo-yo dieting. But, if you decide to do the actions of the Weight Success Method, it'll almost certainly result in you living the rest of your life in your healthy-weight range, and doing so more easily and enjoyably than you ever thought possible. Put simply, it comes down to this.

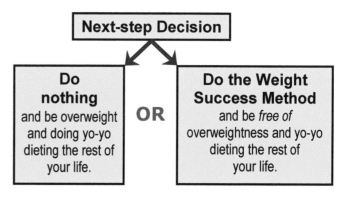

AGAIN — The secret to succeeding at lifelong healthy-weight living is: Do Weight Success Actions <u>every day</u>. You accomplish this by doing the Weight Success Method, which typically takes <u>less than</u> 8 minutes of dedicated time per day.

CHAPTER 4: Attributes of an Ideal Weight Management Program

Weight management programs differ. You deserve the *very best* there is. Here's how to identify it.

IF SOMEONE were to ask me what the attributes should be for an ideal weight management program, I would give them this list of sixteen.

1 – It includes **SUCCESS DRIVERS:** By applying the program one automatically includes most or all of the 19 success drivers in their weight success pursuit and, thereby, overcomes a main reason why many people fail at creating lifelong healthy-weight living — that reason being: Failure to do Weight Success Actions every day.

2 – Is **EASY:** No hard work or deep thought needed. Involves simple daily actions anyone can do in a few minutes per day.

3 – Is **ECONOMICAL:** Fits the budget of ordinary persons.

4 – Is **SAFE:** Doesn't require possibly-risky weird foods or procedures.

5 – Is **HEALTHY:** No radical less-than-fully-healthy eating regimen required. You pursue a dietary program that's healthiest for you.

6 – Is **FLEXIBLE:** No excessive time demands. Can be configured to fit one's daily schedule.

7 – Is **FOCUSED:** Is built on core concepts anyone can remember. Not a collection of cutesy topics with no connecting message.

8 – Is **COMBINABLE:** There's no requirement to adhere to a single dietary approach. Can be combined with any bona fide dietary program of one's choice, including a program of one's own design.

9 – Is **CUSTOMIZABLE:** Doesn't take a "you must do it only this way" approach. Includes all the tools needed for instant, easy startup, but they're all customizable, should one want to tweak any.

10 – Is **ENJOYABLE:** No pain, stress, or inconvenience. Involves activities most persons find enjoyable and gratifying. (For more on this, go to the How the Weight Success Method is Enjoyable chapter, page **123**.)

11 – Is **DUAL-FUNCTION:** Is specially designed to create (a) change achievement that's needed for achieving weight reduction <u>and</u> (b) maintenance achievement that's needed for achieving lifelong healthy-weight living. (For more on this, read The No-change Secret of Maintenance Achievement chapter, page **166**.)

12 – Is **PROVEN:** Has been proved to work, preferably through verification by scientific methodology. But, lacking that, has been proved to work by the creator of the program.

13 – Is **SETBACK APPLICABLE:** Contains a specific procedure for converting any problem or setback into a progress action. (For more on this, read the Setback Reversal Made Easier chapter, page **88**.)

14 – Is **LIFE JOURNEY ENHANCING:** Use of the program expands the basic elements of human flourishing: (1) positive emotions, (2) engagement (a.k.a. flow), (3) positive relationships, (4) meaning, and (5) accomplishment. (For more on this, read the How the Weight Success Method Enhances Your Life Journey chapter, page **157**.)

15 – Is **MINDSET ENHANCING:** Helps a person to build a healthy-weight-promoting mindset (as described in Startup Action 5, page **37**).

16 – Allows for optional **ADVANCED DEVELOPMENT:** Provides a way for those seeking more in-depth knowledge and procedures to get it. (Most of the chapters in Section B are for this purpose. For examples, read the Six More Mind Motivators chapter, page **110**, and the Expanded Weight Success Benefits chapter, page **168**.)

So, which weight management programs come closest to matching this ideal description? I don't know about every program out there. But it's my judgement that the Weight Success Method hits all 16 of the above descriptors. So, the Weight Success Method might not be the only ideal program, but if there are multiple ideal programs, the Weight Success Method is surely one of them.

> Of all the attributes of the Weight Success Method, the most unique and most powerful is: It results in you doing Weight Success Actions <u>every day</u>.

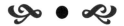

It Comes Down to This

THE EASIEST WAY TO DO
WEIGHT SUCCESS ACTIONS
EVERY DAY IS DO THE
WEIGHT SUCCESS METHOD.

DOING THE METHOD PUTS
SUCCESS DRIVERS
INTO YOUR
WEIGHT SUCCESS PURSUIT,
WHICH CAUSES YOU TO DO
WEIGHT SUCCESS ACTIONS
<u>EVERY</u> DAY,
WHICH RESULTS IN YOU
SUCCEEDING AT CREATING
HEALTHY-WEIGHT LIVING
<u>FOR LIFE</u>.

Weight management comes down to two things: (1) a PROBLEM and (2) a SOLUTION.

WHEN THE world of weight control — a.k.a. weight management — is distilled to its essence it amounts to two main processes. The first process is the dynamic that causes weight gain. We'll label it Problem Process — a.k.a. *overweight* creation process. The second process is the dynamic that causes weight control or the healthy-weight condition. We'll label it Solution Process — a.k.a. *healthy-weight* creation process.

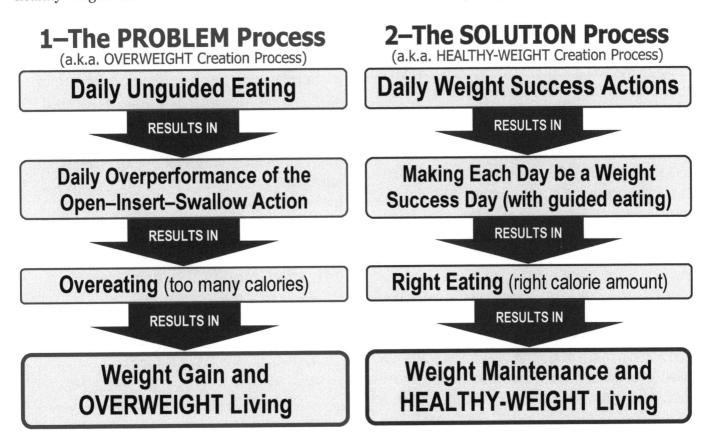

1–The PROBLEM Process
(a.k.a. OVERWEIGHT Creation Process)

Daily Unguided Eating

RESULTS IN

Daily Overperformance of the Open–Insert–Swallow Action

RESULTS IN

Overeating (too many calories)

RESULTS IN

Weight Gain and OVERWEIGHT Living

2–The SOLUTION Process
(a.k.a. HEALTHY-WEIGHT Creation Process)

Daily Weight Success Actions

RESULTS IN

Making Each Day be a Weight Success Day (with guided eating)

RESULTS IN

Right Eating (right calorie amount)

RESULTS IN

Weight Maintenance and HEALTHY-WEIGHT Living

With the thousands of hours and millions of dollars that we've spent in the past 50 years on researching the "zillions" of fat-promoting factors in our world we've adopted the assumption that the cause and cure of overweightness is *COMPLEX.* But in actuality, it's *SIMPLE.* Once society realizes this truth, overweightness will <u>decline</u> and healthy-weight living will <u>ascend</u>.

CHAPTER 6: Healthy-weight Range in Detail

A key factor in creating healthy-weight living is: Identify an achievable healthy-weight *range*.

SOCIETY HAS long overlooked this crucial point: A main cause of our failure to achieve weight management success is we've been defining weight management success in terms of a single number (pound or kilogram). A pound number is a weight target that's just 16 ounces wide. Using a single pound number as one's daily weight target is like having a football goalpost that's 16-inches wide and then defining field goal kicker success in terms of kicking the ball through this ultra-narrow goalpost on every kick. It's so narrow of a target the kicker will miss it on most days. So, for most days the kicker is a *failure*. It's no wonder the pursuit of weight management has been one of the most discouraging endeavors of modern life.

What's the solution? Define weight management success in terms of a weight *range*. By having a weight range as the target it creates the opportunity to be a weight management success every day. I call this range your *healthy-weight range*. I define it as: the weight range that maximizes the likelihood of you living in optimal health. So, your entire healthy-weight range is regarded as being a healthy weight for you. Which means, whenever your body weight is in your healthy-weight range, you're a "weight management *success* who's living at their *healthy weight.*"

Guidelines for Your Healthy-weight Range

There's no one perfect method for setting one's healthy-weight range. But here are some helpful guidelines. Use these and also include your own good judgement. Plus, it could be a good idea to factor in the opinion of a health professional, such as your doctor.

Start by Ascertaining Your Ideal Weight

For the past 150 years the medical profession has created formulas for calculating ideal body weight. These formulas go by various names, typically the name of the inventor. It appears that, at the present time, the most widely accepted formula is the **Robinson formula,** created in 1983.

On the Internet you can find automatic ideal weight calculators based on this formula. You enter your age, gender, and height and it shows an ideal weight number. Here's the URL for one such calculator:

calculator.net/ideal-weight-calculator.html

You'll note that this site also shows the ideal weight derived from some of the other formulas. And you'll further note that all these weights differ from one another. Which tells us that ideal weight calculation isn't an exact science. But, again, the Robinson formula appears to be the one most widely recognized — at the time this book was written — so I suggest going with that one.

If Needed, Modify the Ideal Weight Number to Fit Your Situation

Now here's a major point. If in your opinion the ideal weight number produced by the calculator doesn't fit your situation or won't produce the most effective weight management outcome for you, *adopt whatever ideal weight number you believe will produce the most effective weight management outcome on your weight success journey.* Make sure it's a weight number that's healthy for you. Again, you might find it helpful to factor in the opinion of a physician.

Here are two factors that might warrant changing the ideal weight number produced by the calculator: (a) frame size and (b) muscle mass.

Frame Size. Your frame size — a.k.a. skeletal size or bone size — could be a reason for deviating from the ideal weight number produced by the calculator. The term "frame size" pertains to the width of your bones. Researchers apply three categories to it: small, medium, large — a.k.a. narrow, normal, wide. The weight calculator's number is based on a medium, or normal, frame size. So, generally speaking, if you have a large or wide frame size — sometimes called "big boned" or "large boned" — it might be a good idea to adjust your ideal weight number upward. How much? There's no exact amount, but 10 pounds or more might be called for.

Conversely, if you have a narrow frame size, it might be a good idea to adjust your ideal weight number downward.

So how does one determine whether their frame size is narrow, medium, or wide? There are two ways. One is: measure the circumference of your wrist at the narrowest point. The other is: measure the width of your elbow at the widest point. There's a specific method for doing each. If you're interested in exact instruction, go to the Internet and do a search for "ideal weight based on frame."

Muscle Mass. In addition to being based on normal frame size, the ideal weight calculator is also based on normal muscle size. Which means, if you happen to be genetically endowed with larger than normal muscle size, or if you're a bodybuilder that has acquired extra-large muscles, it might be a good idea to adjust the calculator's ideal weight number upward. How much? That depends on how much larger your muscles are from normal. If you're a bodybuilder with very large muscles, the upward adjustment could be considerable.

Determine How Large Your Healthy-weight Range Span Will Be

So, what should be the size, or span, of your healthy-weight range? I'll begin with this general guideline.

If you weigh in pounds, consider having your healthy-weight range span be either six, seven, or eight pounds.

If you weigh in kilograms, consider having it be either three or four kilos.

But, if you believe an eight pound or a four kilo healthy-weight range is too small for your situation, feel free to expand it slightly to, say, a nine, ten, or eleven pound (or a five kilo) range. Also, if you're a woman who undergoes considerable premenstrual water retention you might find it handy to use a slightly expanded healthy-weight range. That way,

you have ample opportunity to maintain your body weight within your healthy-weight range during the premenstrual period.

In short, consider setting the span of your healthy-weight range to be *about five percent* of your ideal weight number. But, if you have good reason to make it slightly larger or smaller than that, do so.

I'll explain how the "five percent guideline" works. Assume that a person has a 160 pound ideal weight number. Five percent of 160 is eight (0.05 × 160 = 8). So this suggests a healthy-weight range span of eight pounds. Which means, the person would use this 8-pound span number as a starting point and, if necessary, increase or decrease the span from that point to create a healthy-weight range that, in their opinion, will produce the most effective weight management outcome on their weight management journey.

Determine the Upper and Lower Numbers of the Range

So how does one go about setting the high end and low end numbers of their healthy-weight range? There are three ways. Pick the one you believe will work best for you.

WAY #1: *Make Your Ideal Weight the Center Point of the Range.* ✍ For this, have your ideal weight number be near the center of the range, and then build above and below it.

To illustrate, let's assume your ideal weight number is 168 pounds. And, let's further assume you want to have a 7-pound healthy-weight range. To create a 7-pound range around this number you could go three pounds down and three pounds up from 168. This results in a healthy-weight range of 165 to 171 pounds. Which means, any weight within this range (or between 165.0 to 171.9) is considered to be a *healthy weight* for you. So, whenever your body weight is 165, 166, 167, 168, 169, 170, or 171 pounds (or between 165.0–171.9 lbs.) you're living at your healthy weight.

And what about kilograms? If your ideal weight number happened to be 76 kilos and you wanted a 3-kilo healthy-weight range, you could go one kilo down and one kilo up from 76, thereby creating a healthy-weight range of 75 to 77 kilos. So, any weight between 75.0–77.9 kilos would be considered to be a healthy weight for you.

WAY #2: *Make Your Ideal Weight Number the Lower Limit of the Range.* ❧ For this, have your ideal weight number be the bottom point of the range, and then build upward from there.

To illustrate, let's assume once again your ideal weight number is 168 pounds. And, let's further assume you want to have a 7-pound healthy-weight range. To create a healthy-weight range with this number at the bottom you would go six pounds up from 168. This results in a healthy-weight range of 168 to 174 pounds. Which means, any weight within this range (or between 168.0 to 174.9) is considered to be a *healthy weight* for you. So, whenever your body weight is 168, 169, 170, 171, 172, 173, or 174 pounds (or between 168.0–174.9 lbs.) you're living at your healthy weight.

And what about kilograms? If your ideal weight number happened to be 76 kilos and you wanted a 3-kilo healthy-weight range with your ideal weight at the bottom, you would go two kilos up from 76, thereby creating a healthy-weight range of 76 to 78 kilos. So, any weight between 76.0–78.9 kilos would be considered to be a healthy weight for you.

WAY #3: *Make Your Ideal Weight Number the Upper Limit of the Range.* ❧ For this, have your ideal weight number be the top point of the range, and then build downward from there. The procedure for this is the same as for doing Way #2 (above), except in the opposite direction.

So, which of these three ways is best for you? I suggest you use whichever one you believe will produce the most effective weight management outcome for you.

Your Ideal Weight and Healthy-weight Range Can Change Over Time

Evolving conditions can warrant a change in ideal weight number and healthy-weight range. For example, if you're growing taller your ideal weight and healthy-weight range will likely move upward.

And, if your muscle mass is shrinking, as happens to most persons after about age 35 or 40, your ideal weight and weight range will likely move downward. Also, as you grow older your ideal weight goes down. So, as your age, height, and amount of muscle mass changes, you should adjust your healthy-weight range accordingly. And, you should reflect this in your Weight Success Benefits Directive (p. 52) by changing your healthy-weight range numbers.

Closing Comment and Warning

In setting your ideal weight number, bear this point in mind: Good health is always more important than "good looks." Meaning, don't be tempted into pursuing a super-low, or ultra-thin, ideal weight number just because you, or friends or family, think you look "good" or "sexy" at that weight. Conversely, don't be seduced into keeping your body weight in the overweight range just because you, or friends or family, think you look "good" or "strong" or "healthy" at that weight. Living overweight increases the likelihood of incurring any of numerous debilitating conditions. Ditto for living underweight. In short, there's nothing good-looking, healthy, or sexy about being the victim of some debilitating illness caused by living overweight or underweight.

Also, you'll likely discover that most people don't know what constitutes healthy body weight. What they view as an ideal or healthy weight is about 25 pounds higher than an actual ideal body weight. Which means, if you rely on what other people think is the "right weight" for you, you'll likely end up being about 25 pounds *overweight,* or 25 pounds beyond your ideal or healthiest weight.

Why do most people carry this distorted view? It's because, in our world correct weight is the *exception,* overweightness is the *rule.* We're removed from the womb by overweight doctors and nurses. We grow up playing with overweight friends. We're raised by overweight parents. We're taught by overweight teachers, coaches, and role models. The result: We automatically view the overweight body as being the norm and view the correct weight body as an underweight "ab-norm."

To illustrate, here's a story. Shortly after starting the Weight Success Method in 2007 I moved my weight down some pounds, to live in what I figured was my healthy-weight range. This change prompted a family member to occasionally tell me "you're too skinny," "you need to put on some pounds," and so on. Finally, I decided action was in order. I did some Internet research to find out exactly what my ideal weight number was. As it turned out, depending on how it was calculated I was either right at my ideal weight or *slightly above* it. I typed up my findings and gave copies to family members. The comments on my body weight came no more.

It's about Living in the Right Range

View it this way. You have an overall possible body weight range that consists of three parts: underweight range, healthy-weight range, overweight range. Make sure you live your life in the one that produces greatest health benefit. As an infographic it looks like this.

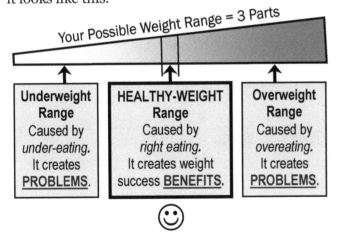

Did You Know ...

Research indicates that when we're living <u>non</u>-overweight, or at our ideal weight, the likelihood of us living FREE OF a major affliction is *much greater* than when we're living overweight. Here's a list of the bad situa-

tions that <u>non</u>-overweight living helps a person to <u>avoid</u>: high blood pressure • high blood cholesterol • congestive heart failure • heart attack • blood clots in legs and lungs • stroke • gout • Alzheimer's disease • osteoarthritis • type 2 diabetes • colon cancer • breast cancer • uterine cancer (women) • prostate cancer (men) • liver cirrhosis • gallstones and gall bladder disorders • sleeping disorders such as sleep apnea and excessive snoring • joint and lower back problems • infertility • incontinence • menstrual problems and pregnancy issues • and psychological disorders such as depression and lowered self-esteem.

Weight Success Days
are the Building Blocks of lifelong Healthy-weight Living, and the Weight Success Method is the easiest way to create Weight Success Days.

Doing
Weight Success Actions
every day is the Way to
Lifelong Weight Success

CHAPTER 7: Weight Success Benefits in Detail

Once you fully identify and then daily visualize the benefits of healthy-weight living and weight success, self-motivation becomes *easier.*

TO MAXIMIZE the likelihood of creating lifelong heathy-weight living, you must clearly identify your weight success benefits. Then reflect on these benefits each day. By doing this it motivates your mind to pursue activities that result in realizing these benefits, which includes the activity of creating lifelong healthy-weight living. Here's how to identify your weight success benefits.

Create a list of the good things that will come your way from living in your healthy-weight range. We call these good things *weight success benefits.* To make your benefits listing job easy I've included a list of 20 possible benefits (coming up below). Of course, *you should ignore those that don't apply to you.* Plus you should add in any benefit that does apply but isn't on the list. Your final list can include both general benefits and specific. Use whatever wording carries the most meaning for you.

20 Possible Benefits from Living in Your Healthy-weight Range

1. I have a greater chance of *living healthier longer* — or greater chance of living free of debilitating accidents, illnesses, diseases, and bodily malfunction.
2. I experience greater eating pleasure.
3. I feel better.
4. I look better.
5. I move better.
6. I have greater agility.
7. I have greater energy and stamina.
8. I experience greater happiness, including a daily good feeling from creating lifelong healthy-weight living.
9. I have a stronger self-image and enhanced self-esteem.
10. I have better overall health and fewer annoying ailments.
11. My clothes fit better and feel more comfortable.
12. I'm no longer constantly growing out of clothes.
13. I can do more [of a particular fun thing or things].
14. I eliminate [a particular illness or affliction].
15. I improve [a particular relationship].
16. I overcome [a particular problem].
17. I can better engage in [a particular activity or pursuit].
18. I have a greater chance of avoiding debilitating physical accidents, such as broken bones from falling.
19. I have a greater chance of living longer.
20. I will be more active in my latter years.

Write down your list of weight success benefits in the Benefits section of the Weight Success Benefits Directive (p. **52**). Note: Don't assume that the prior list of 20 benefits includes every possible weight success benefit. There may be additional benefits not on this list, which you might want to include.

REPEAT: Write It Down!

Either (a) *write down* or (b) *type up and print out* your list of weight success benefits. Then insert this list into your Weight Success Benefits Directive (p. 52), which you use in Daily Action 3.

Be Sure to Include Benefit #1

You can include whatever benefits you want in your weight success benefits list. But I suggest you be sure to include Benefit #1 (shown in prior list). That benefit is: a greater chance of living healthier longer — or greater chance of living free of debilitating accidents, illnesses, diseases, and bodily malfunction.

Perhaps you're wondering why Benefit #1 is Number One. It's because as a person ages the chance of contracting a debilitating affliction increases substantially. Research shows that when you're living <u>non</u>-overweight the likelihood of you living FREE OF a major affliction is much greater than when you're living overweight. Here's a list of the bad situations that <u>non</u>-overweight living helps a person to <u>avoid</u>: high blood pressure • high blood cholesterol • congestive heart failure • heart attack • blood clots in legs and lungs • stroke • gout • Alzheimer's disease • osteoarthritis • type 2 diabetes • colon cancer • breast cancer • uterine cancer (women) • prostate cancer (men) • liver cirrhosis • gallstones and gall bladder disorders • sleeping disorders such as sleep apnea and excessive snoring • joint and lower back problems • infertility • incontinence • menstrual problems and pregnancy issues • and psychological disorders such as depression and lowered self-esteem.

Increasing the likelihood of living FREE OF those conditions is a high priority to many folks, which is why "a greater chance of living healthier longer" is the #1 weight success benefit.

TO CONCLUDE, each day read your weight success benefits list and visualize at least one of the benefits as an accomplished fact. Generate a good feeling from the visualization. This motivates your mind — especially your subconscious mind — to create thoughts and feelings that guide you toward creation of that benefit, which will involve creation of healthy-weight living.

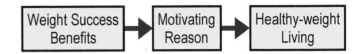

A Final Big Reason

Here's one more reason for living your life in your healthy-weight range. Many of us express how much we love and care for our children, grandchildren, and other family members. But I suggest, also include this action: *Live the rest of your life in your healthy-weight range.* Doing so is one of the truest love expressions of all, in two ways.

First, by living the rest of your life in your healthy-weight range you provide family members with an inspiring role model to emulate — a role model of healthy-weight living. The result: at least some will follow your example, which will cause them to live a healthier, happier, more fulfilling life.

Second, by living in your healthy-weight range you greatly *reduce* the chance of you contracting a debilitating condition as a result of extended overweight living. This, in turn, reduces the likelihood of your children or other family members having to bear the crushing responsibility of looking after you for years while you're living out your life in an incapacitated state.

Indeed, living the rest of your life in your healthy-weight range is one of the most loving, caring, thoughtful things you can do for those who are nearest and dearest to you. So, engaging in healthy-weight living isn't merely an act of self-development and personal achievement. It goes way beyond that.

Healthy-weight living provides a plethora of benefits — way more than most persons imagine it to be. Perhaps the greatest benefit of all is having a greater chance of *living healthier longer.*

CHAPTER 8: Weighing and Scale Info

A consistently accurate bathroom scale, *properly* used each day, is the most powerful tool on the planet for creating healthy-weight living.

YOU MIGHT find this hard to believe, but it's true. Correct daily weighing (Daily Action 1) combined with a certain right response (Daily Action 2A or 2B) is the core element to creating lifelong healthy-weight living. So, you need a scale that delivers a consistently accurate weight reading every time. If you already have such a scale, great. But, if you don't have a consistently accurate scale it would likely be a good idea to get one.

Contrary to what you might assume, many bathroom scales do *not* produce a consistently accurate weight reading. Meaning, if you step on the scale two times in a row you'll get two different readings — sometimes as much as two or three pounds (or a kilo) apart. This type of scale doesn't best serve our purpose.

Also contrary to what you might assume, there seems to be no correlation between a bathroom scale's accuracy and its stylishness, size, type, or price. Meaning, a fancy stylish scale will deliver an inaccurate or inconsistent reading as often as a plain-looking scale — a big scale will deliver an inaccurate or inconsistent reading as often as a smaller scale — a digital (electronic sensor) scale will deliver an inaccurate or inconsistent reading as often as a mechanical (spring) scale — and an expensive bathroom scale will deliver an inaccurate or inconsistent reading as often as a lower-priced scale.

If you don't believe it, do as I did. Go to the scale section of a well-stocked bathroom supplies store — like, for example, Bed Bath & Beyond — and conduct a test. Weigh yourself on the various sample test models. With each one, stand on it three times in a row. I predict you'll find the inconsistency to be eye-opening.

Finally, as a result of your testing, get the best-performing scale your budget will allow. By "best-performing scale" I mean the scale that comes

closest to delivering a *consistently accurate* weight reading for you.

Eventually, I did some Internet research and ended up buying a type of scale used in most doctors' offices. Such a scale typically comes in two types: (a) a high-end digital scale and (b) a balance beam, or weigh beam, scale. The weigh beam scale is the traditional type of scale that has been used in doctors' offices for about the past century or so. It's the one that looks like a giant "T" and has a weigh bar with a sliding weight at the top of the "T", as depicted in this Microsoft clipart sketch.

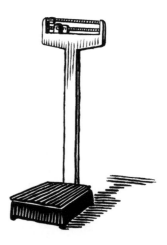

The digital scale, on the other hand, is more recent. It's slick looking and gives an instant reading. But it can be somewhat pricey. You might find that a "home version" of the weigh beam scale carries a more reasonable price tag.

My personal preference is the weigh beam, not just because of its lower price but because I like the way it works. I like sliding the weigh bar weight to the proper spot. Plus, it doesn't require batteries or electric cords. Plus, because of its tall height I see it many times each day, which makes it a reminder to do the five daily actions.

TIP 1: If you happen to get a weigh beam scale here's a handy suggestion. Each time after getting onto the scale <u>or</u> after sliding the weigh-bar weight, slightly raise your arms up and down a little bit. Do this just once. This "jiggles" the weigh beam, which causes it to instantly move to a new correct position. You might find that you do this "arm jiggle" movement several times during a weighing (each time after adjusting the weigh beam), in order to ascertain the final correct weight in that weighing.

TIP 2: After many years of using the weigh beam scale I wanted to achieve a more precise weighing, or smaller opening where the "needle" floats to indicate a weight reading. To do that, I cut a small piece of aluminum bar and bolted it to the scale to reduce the size of the opening. Here's a photo that illustrates.

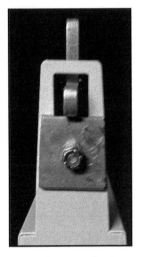

Moving on, several manufacturers make doctor's office scales. Some produce a broad line of both digital scales and weigh beam scales. The scale I personally use, for example, is the *Detecto physician weigh beam scale model 437* — website: detecto.com. It runs about $150 (in 2013). This might seem like a lot of money for a scale. But likely it will last a lifetime. So, what's the annualized cost? If, say, you use it for 20 years, the cost amounts to about $7.50 per year ($150 ÷ 20 = $7.50 per year), or just two cents a day. It's sold through various online sellers including amazon.com. Also, should you happen to get this scale you might like to know that the company has an operating manual titled "Trouble Shooting Guide for Detecto Mechanical Physicians Balance Beam Scales." They will email it upon request.

Important Final Note on Scales
I've mentioned the above-cited specific scale model to provide possibly helpful info. This is <u>not</u> a product promotion or endorsement. There are a number of good scales that can do the job. I've opted for a balance beam scale because it fits my personal preferences. <u>But</u> you might find that a *digital* scale best fits *your* preferences. ***You should get the type and brand of scale that, in your opinion, will work best for YOU and YOUR SITUATION.***

* * *

– "2B or Not 2B" –
Two Opposite Approaches

There are two opposing approaches to solving the worldwide overweight problem. They work like this.

APPROACH #1: We continue doing those "cause of our overweightness" or "fat-promoting factors" studies that tell us we humans have no control over how much we eat and weigh. (For a listing of fat-promoting factors, go to "False Assumption 1" in the 16 False Assumptions that Are Sabotaging Us chapter, page 146.)

APPROACH #2: Everyone go on a diet and take their weight down to their healthy-weight range; then weigh themselves each day and whenever their daily weight reading goes above their healthy-weight range they enact a Weight Correction Day of total fasting or semi-fasting and, so, bring their weight back into their healthy-weight range in 24–48 hours. (See Daily Action 2B, page 48.)

The first approach will continue costing millions and solve nothing. The second would cost virtually nothing and solve the worldwide overweight problem in a year. Here's how it's expressed as an infographic (next page).

Two approaches to pursuing Healthy-weight Living:
Which One Will We Opt For?

APPROACH #1
Continue fruitlessly pursuing research based on the erroneous notion that there are fat-promoting factors beyond individual human control which are forcing each of us and society-at-large to live in a state of overweightness.

OR

APPROACH #2
Pursue the concept of each person (a) enacting a weight management program that takes them to their healthy-weight range, then (b) weighing themself each day and anytime their weight goes above their healthy-weight range immediately enact a Weight Correction Day that brings their weight back into their healthy-weight range in 24–48 hours.

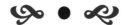

There's a driving dynamic in the world of weight management and healthy-weight living — it's **Calorie Consumption.**
It works like this — <u>remember it</u>.

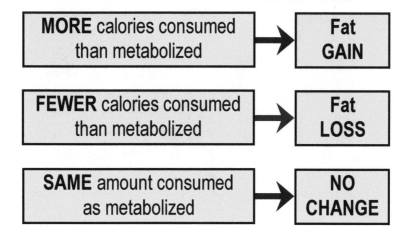

MORE calories consumed than metabolized	Fat **GAIN**
FEWER calories consumed than metabolized	Fat **LOSS**
SAME amount consumed as metabolized	**NO CHANGE**

CHAPTER 9: Detailed Instructions for Weight Success Benefits Directive

Apply these simple instructions for setting up and delivering the Weight Success Benefits Directive (p. 52) and you'll greatly magnify the positive impact of the Directive.

TO GET maximum results from your Weight Success Benefits Directive you need to do three things: (1) fill in the blank sections of the Directive, (2) enhance the Directive, if needed, and (3) deliver the Directive in a way that produces maximum effect. The next three sections tell how to do those three things.

1 - Filling in the Blanks

The Weight Success Benefits Directive contains three blank line (_____) sections. TIP: For filling in these blanks I suggest you use a pencil, not a pen. Here's how to do it.

Healthy-weight Range

In the first two blanks insert your desired healthy-weight range in either pounds or kilos. Your healthy-weight range should be a *bona fide* healthy-weight range for your gender, height, and age. For the "pounds–kilos" phrase draw a line through the word that doesn't apply. For explanation of how to set your healthy-weight range, go to the *Healthy-weight Range in Detail* chapter (p. **76**).

Preferred Dietary Program

In the next blank insert the name of your preferred dietary program. I define *preferred dietary program* as a set of eating guidelines and eating practices you prefer to follow and which, when followed, lead you to good health and healthy-weight living. Another name for preferred dietary program is preferred eating strategy.

So, if you're presently in weight reduction pursuit, then whatever eating program you're pursuing for your diet, weight loss, or weight reduction program is what you specify as your "preferred dietary program" in the Weight Success Benefits Directive. After you go into weight mainte-nance pursuit, you then specify the maintenance eating program you'll be following for staying in your healthy-weight range.

Your preferred dietary program can be any bona fide dietary program presently on the market or it can be a program of your own design. For more info on identifying a preferred dietary program, read Startup Action 7 (p. **40**). If you think you might want to create a program of your own design, I suggest you first read the *Author's Approach to Eating* chapter (p. **94**).

Weight Success Benefits

In the last blank section — which consists of a set of lines — insert a listing of the benefits you'll derive from living in your healthy-weight range. For help in defining your weight success benefits, I suggest reading the *Weight Success Benefits in Detail* chapter (p. **80**).

The Weight Success Benefits Directive contains about 20 lines for listing weight success benefits. You're not required to fill every line. Some people have just three or four weight success benefits. Others have a dozen or more.

To install your list into the Directive you can either write it in or type it up and tape it in. If you write it in I suggest using a pencil.

As you already know, you'll be reading your Weight Success Benefits Directive each day. If your weight success benefits list is a lengthy one it will add an extra minute or so of reading time. But if it happens you'd like to keep reading time to a minimum, here's an optional tactic to consider. Divide your weight success benefits list into seven groups. Assign each group to a particular day of the week. Then, each day when reading the Directive, read the group of benefits assigned to that day, and overlook reading the other six groups on that day.

2 – Enhancing the Directive, If Needed

The Weight Success Benefits Directive isn't carved in granite; instead it's a changeable document. So, if there's something you'd like to delete, draw a line through it. If there's something you'd like to change, draw a line through it and write the new word or words above.

Reading the Directive the first few times might seem like work. But, after a few days it begins to become enjoyable, even fun. This especially occurs when results start happening, which is almost immediately.

3 – Seven Actions for Delivering the Directive for Maximum Effect

To maximize the results you get from the Weight Success Benefits Directive, apply these seven actions when delivering it. (Note: You can advantageously apply these actions to delivery of any mind directive, not just this directive.)

1 – Speak it. ❧ Speaking aloud is best, but when you can't do that, whisper it to yourself. As you whisper it make your tongue and lips move. (Note: You can convey directives to your mind by speaking silently in your mind. But, for the Weight Success Benefits Directive I recommend that you speak it aloud or at least whisper it.)

2 – Act as-if your mind is a *distinct being* that's listening to every instruction you're giving it. ❧ (For more about your mind, go to the Why the Weight Success Method Gets Your Whole Mind Involved chapter, page **129**.)

3 – Use some emotional force. ❧ That is, put some passion or emotional intensity into the delivery. Note: Happiness and excitement are forms of emotional intensity.

4 – Hold a strong desire for your mind to do every action described in the Directive. ❧ The stronger you desire for your mind to perform the actions described in the Directive, the more important these actions appear to your mind — including subconscious mind. And, the more

important these actions appear to your mind, the more diligently it strives to do them.

So, how do you strengthen your desire for your mind to do what's called for in the Weight Success Benefits Directive? You imagine how good you'll feel and how great your life will be from gaining the benefits of maintaining your weight in your healthy-weight range. These benefits, by the way, are the items you list in the Weight Success Benefits section of the Directive. The more vividly you imagine how good you'll feel from deriving these benefits, the more diligently your mind — especially your subconscious mind — will pursue actualization of the benefits.

5 – Hold the belief that your mind can and will perform the actions. ❧ Hold this belief not only while delivering the Directive but afterward, as well. This is vital. When you hold doubt, or halfway belief, that your mind will do the actions described in a request or directive it creates a problem. It causes your mind to ignore doing the actions. This happens because your mind seldom performs in contradiction to the belief system held in your mind. So, when you hold the belief "I can't do action X" or "my mind won't do action X" or "action X is impossible to do," your mind — including your subconscious mind — will respond accordingly. As a result, it likely won't perform the actions described in the Directive.

So, how do you replace disbelief with belief? You make-believe, or act as-if, you believe. That's right, you totally pretend you're holding the belief that you — or your mind — can and will perform the actions described in the Weight Success Benefits Directive. I realize this instruction might sound hokey. But do it anyhow; it works. For more on this, see the *How Believing and Acting As-if Work* section, page **38**.

6 – Visualize one or more of your weight success benefits as an accomplished fact. ❧ After reading the list of weight success benefits take 30 seconds to visualize, or imagine, yourself at that very moment enjoying having at least one of the exciting benefits.

7 – Apply **creative delivery techniques** for extra effect. ❧ Doing this can cause your mind to pay extra attention to what you're telling it to do. Here are some examples to consider.

FIRST, emphasize the key words. You can do this by speaking slightly louder, or slower, or more forcefully. These key words are printed in *italic,* <u>underline</u>, or **bold.**

SECOND, repeat (reread) a particular phrase or sentence for emphasis.

THIRD, read the entire Directive slowly and deliberately. This will require one or two extra minutes. But it can pay dividends. It can cause your subconscious mind to pay special attention to the instructions contained in the Directive. To do this, pause for a few seconds after each sentence. During the pause, reflect on the meaning or main message of the sentence.

FOURTH, ad lib whenever you see fit. Insert spontaneous additional instructions to your subconscious mind to emphasize key points.

FIFTH, deliver the Directive in a different place or position. For example, if you've been delivering the Directive sitting down, do it standing. Or, deliver it while pacing, like you're delivering a speech. Include arm movement and gesticulation of main points. This can be a powerful form of delivery. It can enhance your emotional impact. Experiment and find out what works best for you. Or, just change delivery style from time to time for variety.

> To sum up, the Weight Success Benefits Directive is an *important* message for your mind. Deliver it like it is and your mind — especially your subconscious mind — will act accordingly.

Right-eating mindset creates right-eating actions which create right-weight living. Yes, mindset <u>is</u> the key.

Mindset → causes → **Actions** → causes → **Weight**

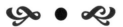

Do
Weight Success Actions
EVERY DAY

CHAPTER 10: Setback Reversal Made Easier

In every endeavor, challenges and setbacks happen. Succeeding at an endeavor requires converting setbacks into progress actions. Those who do this, succeed. Those who don't, fail or quit.

WITH ALMOST every pursuit a person can accidentally deviate from the program now and then. So, on your weight success journey you might now and then forget to do what you want to be doing and, instead, accidentally engage in wrong eating. I call this a *misstep* — also known as accidental oversight. Here's an example. A special meal comes along and you become caught up in the moment and, thereby, overlook doing the Guided Eating Process (of Daily Action 5 of the Weight Success Method) and you end up accidentally overeating.

Here's another example of a misstep. An old overeating-causing habit or craving that you've shut down now temporarily reactivates during a certain meal or on a certain day. You unthinkingly respond to this temporarily reactivated habit or craving the wrong way — that is, by eating too much — and this results in overeating for the day.

Also, with every endeavor there are periods when progress seems to stop. For example, when striving to lose weight, weight loss might stop. Or, when living in your healthy-weight range, a jump in weight that takes you outside the range might occur. I call this a *progress lapse*.

In both these situations — misstep and progress lapse — you should apply the same response: Immediately turn the setback into a progress action. You can easily do this by applying a certain set of actions. I call it the *setback-reversal process*. It involves six actions plus an optional seventh action. Here now is how to do the setback-reversal process, which is the easiest way to create a progress action out of a misstep or progress lapse.

ACTION 1: Avoid a counterproductive response and adopt a productive one.

This is Action 1 because if you don't do this nothing else works, or works well. Examples of a counter-

productive response include second-guessing, self-doubt, self-pity, self-blame, guilt, and discouragement. These things never help and usually hurt. They make it harder to create a timely correction or reversal of the misstep or progress lapse. So, avoid every type of counterproductive response. Instead, adopt the attitude "What has happened is over; I'm now going to *learn* and *benefit* from it." In short, shun negative responses; embrace a positive one.

ACTION 2: Identify the cause.

The next step to creating a progress action out of a misstep or progress lapse is identify the cause. The cause of most missteps and progress lapses is a failure to remember to do what you needed to be doing. Or, in short, a failure to apply all five daily actions of the Weight Success Method each day.

ACTION 3: Identify the future corrective action.

For this step you identify the specific corrective action you'll be taking in the future to avert a repeat of the misstep or progress lapse. Basically, what you want to be doing next time is take the opposite action to whatever action caused the misstep.

For example, let's assume the misstep was caused by you forgetting to do the Guided Eating Process (p. **56**) during a meal. In this case, next time a similar situation arises the corrective action would be for you to remember to do the Guided Eating Process during the meal.

ACTION 4: Deliver a misstep-reversal directive.

Deliver a mini directive to your self — or your mind — that orders it to apply the corrective action the next time you encounter the type of situation that resulted in the past misstep or progress lapse. Here's how it might go.

Subconscious mind, the next time I encounter [the situation that resulted in the misstep], you are to remind me to [take such-and-such corrective action]. I <u>strongly desire</u> for you to do this and I <u>firmly believe</u> you will do so. Working together, we <u>will</u> convert the past misstep into a progress action, and <u>will</u> avoid the misstep happening again. I greatly appreciate your help in this, and I thank you for it.

> ### ACTION 5: Deliver your Healthy-weight Goal Statement 100 times.

Yes, you read it right. Say your Healthy-weight Goal Statement 100 times. You can either do this aloud, including in a whisper, or do it silently in your mind. Do it within 24 hours after the misstep. You need not do it all in one session. You can spread it out over the 24-hour period if you like.

Does repeating the Statement 100 times seem like a lot? Well, it's not. You're able to say it three times in 12 to 15 seconds. That's 12 to 15 times a minute. Which means, you can do it 100 times in less than eight minutes. If you prefer, you can break it up into two or more sessions. And, you can do them in bed when going to sleep and when you awaken in the morning, and during all the numerous "free time" periods in your day. For more info see the "How to Do It" section (p. **54**) in Daily Action 4.

> ### ACTION 6: Make certain you're doing all five Daily Actions, in entirety, each day.

My personal experience has been this. Whenever I've had a misstep or progress lapse — which, by the way, is very infrequently any more — it has occurred during a brief period when I had been "slacking off" on doing all five daily actions of the Weight Success Method each day.

Also, it has been my further experience that most of my progress lapses occurred on days when

I had been involved in an "extra-tempting meal" situation and had forgotten to do Daily Action 5 (Guided Eating) during that meal. If it happens that this is the situation with your present misstep or progress lapse, do this. For the next seven days deliver this backup depiction statement to yourself at least 10 times each day.

I am right now in a guided-eating week. I do guided eating every time I eat.

Again, say it at least 10 times each day for a week. If you need to refresh yourself on the 3-step Guided Eating Process, go to page **56** in the Daily Action 5 section.

> ### OPTIONAL ACTION 7: Squelch recurring undesired weight readings.

Are you presently experiencing too many days of "undesired-weight readings," or too many recurring days of gaining weight or going over your healthy-weight range? If so, in addition to doing Actions 1–6 also do this Action 7. It involves these three steps.

1. Check your healthy-weight *commitment.* ✍ Is living in your healthy-weight range a *mandatory*, <u>non</u>-optional, <u>will</u>-do, <u>must</u>-have aspect of your life? If it's not, make the firm decision — right now — that it will be for the rest of your life, and remember this decision *each day.*

2. Check your healthy-weight *beliefs.* ✍ Are you holding can-do, will-do beliefs as regards living in your healthy-weight range? Each day are you acting on the assumption that living in your healthy-weight range is, or can be, *easily* doable by you? If you're not doing this, or are finding it hard to do, read the *How Believing and Acting As-if Work* section (p. **38**) in Startup Action 5. Then apply those instructions, including the part about each day *acting as-if* you possess the capability to easily live your life in your healthy-weight range. Also, when doing Daily Actions 3 and 4, be sure to believe and act as-if what they describe is actually happening.

3. Increase your right-eating *focus* and *communication.* ✍ No matter how many "undesired-weight days" you might be experiencing, no

matter how much you might be struggling with overeating, no matter what fat-promoting factor you might be confronting, there's an amount of focus and communication that will reverse the situation. So your job is this: Ratchet up your right-eating focus and right-eating communication to the point it *overpowers* the situation that's making it hard for you to be free of frequently-recurring undesired weight readings. The rest of this chapter explains how to do this.

How to Increase Right-eating FOCUS and COMMUNICATION

The first essential condition to overcoming a situation of recurring undesired weight readings is to ratchet up your right-eating resolve. The way to do this is: Make the resolute decision to immediately begin reversing the situation, *starting that day*. Then deliver a right-eating directive to your mind. Tell it how much you desire to be doing daily right eating and living your life in your healthy-weight range. Describe how doing this will greatly benefit you and your life. And, deliver this communication with vehemence. Lastly, increase your commitment to doing all five daily actions of the Weight Success Method, in entirety, *every day*.

The second essential condition to overcoming a situation of recurring undesired weight readings is to increase right-eating communication to your mind — including subconscious mind. You have three options for doing this, cleverly called Options 1, 2, and 3. Select the one you'd like to do.

Option #1 (p. **90**) involves doing an expanded version of the five daily actions of the Weight Success Method. It's the simplest option of the three.

Option #2 (p. **91**) involves adding a new mind motivator to the five daily actions. You have a choice of six new motivators. The *Six More Mind Motivators* chapter (p. **110**) describes them. This option is a bit more complex than Option 1, but you might find it more powerful.

Option #3 (p. **91**) — which I call *High-power Eat-right Solution* — involves a set of seven specific

actions. It's an all-in, pedal-to-the-metal technique aimed at squelching creeping weight gain, or ending recurring overeating progress lapses. It's the most complex of the three options, but you'll likely find it the most powerful.

So, which option should you do? Do whichever one you think will work best. If you're not sure, you might start with Option #1. If it does the job, stick with it. If it doesn't, do Option #2. If #2 works — great. If it doesn't, do Option #3.

It's virtually certain at least one of these three options will result in you conquering whatever situation is causing your recurring overeating missteps or weight gain progress lapses. But always bear in mind, regardless of which option you choose, the key to success is: *Increase* the amount of right-eating focus and right-eating communication to the point it overwhelms, or conquers, the weight-gain-causing overeating. I call this the "Overeating-reversal Dynamic." Here's the infographic.

Overeating-reversal Works Like This

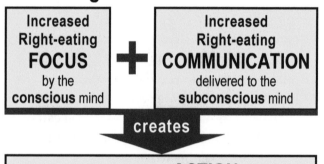

Right-eating FOCUS = Time spent thinking about, talking about, pursuing, and enjoyably doing right eating and healthy-weight living.

Right-eating COMMUNICATION = Communication that tells your mind to steer you toward right eating and healthy-weight living.

Option #1:
Expand the Five Daily Actions

Setback reversal often boils down to doing the daily actions of the Weight Success Method with greater frequency and intensity. Here are some ways to do that. You can use just one way or you can use more than one — your choice.

In Daily Action 2A, increase the emotional intensity, or exuberance, you use when delivering the Thank You, Keep It Up message.

In Daily Action 3, enhance the delivery of your Weight Success Benefits Directive to increase its motivating impact on your mind. See the "Seven Actions for Delivering the Directive for Maximum Effect" section, page **86**, for ways you can enhance delivery.

In Daily Action 4, increase the number of times you say your Healthy-weight Goal Statement throughout the day. And, say it with increased passion. Also, make sure you say it *every* time you begin eating.

In Daily Action 5, increase the amount of guided-eating self-talk during eating sessions. This includes both the number of times you say your Healthy-weight Goal Statement and also the amount of ad lib self-talk. For more on this see the During-eating Self-talk section (p. **59**) in Daily Action 5. Plus, make sure you're holding the belief and acting as-if your mind is right then in the process of doing what's described in your Weight Success Benefits Directive. And, when doing this be on the lookout for a stop-eating signal. (A listing of possible stop-eating signals is given on page **58** in Daily Action 5.) Finally, when the stop-eating signal comes, follow it immediately and also thank your subconscious mind for sending it.

Option #2:
Include Optional Mind Motivators

Would you like to test some additional ways of motivating your mind to assist with creating right eating and healthy-weight living? These techniques are powerful. Plus they can be fun.

Go to the *Six More Mind Motivators* chapter (p. **110**) and check out the optional six mind motivators. Choose the one that looks most promising and give it a try. If it works, do it each day along with the five daily actions. If it doesn't work, try another one of the six optional motivators. Note: You can do more than one a day, if you like. The more you do, the greater the impact.

Option #3:
Do the High-power Eat-right Solution

You use this High-power Eat-right Solution along with the Weight Success Method, not in place of it. It's an all-in, super-powerful, pedal-to-the-metal fix for preventing recurring weight gain and also creeping weight gain. You can use it one or both of two ways.

Firstly, as previously explained, you can use it for this optional Action 7 of the setback-reversal process. Secondly, you can, if you like, use it whenever you confront a day that holds high potential for overeating. I'm talking about those days that contain extra-tempting food and a lot of it — like social events, picnics, parties, weddings, religious celebration days, Thanksgiving, and the like.

Now that you know *when* to use the Solution, here's *how* to do it. It involves seven actions.

ACTION 1: *Recognize the real cause of weight gain.* Bear in mind that weight gain comes from consuming more metabolizable calories than what your body is metabolizing, or "burning up," per day — called *overeating.*

Further, bear in mind that small daily amounts of overeating create small daily amounts of weight gain. So, to avoid creeping weight gain, avoid over-eating even in small daily amounts. For more on this, go to Startup Action 1, page **35**.

ACTION 2: *Realize that right eating is the fix for recurring weight gain.* Or, put another way, realize that to end recurring or creeping weight gain you must end daily overeating, even in small amounts, and install right eating in its place. *Right eating* is the act of eating right foods in right amounts and doing it in a way that creates right eating enjoyment. For more, go to Startup Action 6 (p. **39**).

ACTION 3: *Define your daily maximum calorie allotment number.* For each day you're using this Solution, define the maximum number of daily calories you want to be consuming for that day. If it happens that your preferred dietary program specifies certain types of food you should be eating, then determine what amounts of these foods will equate with your daily maximum calorie allotment number.

Note: This number is not a wish-for number or a nice-to-attain number; it's a *firm, fixed, must-not-exceed* number. Consuming a little less than the daily calorie allotment number is okay, but consuming more is absolutely forbidden. So, do <u>not</u> exceed your daily calorie allotment number for the day.

To make it easier, you might divide the daily calorie allotment number into either meal calorie allotments or day-part calorie allotments. For example, if your daily calorie allotment is, say, 1000 calories, you might assign 200 calories to the breakfast meal, 200 calories to lunch, and 600 calories to dinner. Or, if you use the day-part approach, you might assign 200 calories to the 7 a.m. to noon part, 200 calories to the noon to 4:00 p.m. part, and 600 calories to the 4:00 to 7:00 p.m. part. Note: this amount and distribution of calories is an example, not a recommendation.

Then, every time you eat something, record what you ate and the number of calories consumed from that particular food. Keep a running total for the day, to ensure you don't go over your daily calorie allotment.

Or, if you like, for ultimate simplicity create an eating menu or plan covering the entire day. Specify the exact foods you're going to eat, the exact portion amount of each item, and the number of calories in each item. Set the portion amounts so the total number of calories equals your daily calorie allotment. Then eat exactly what the menu specifies, and no more.

ACTION 4: *Create and hold a weight success mindset.* ✏ Having such a mindset is vital to achieving sustained right eating and healthy-weight living. To create a weight success mindset hold these two assumptions in mind:

1. "Doing right eating and living in my healthy-weight range is a *mandatory* feature of my

existence. It's a <u>non</u>-optional, <u>will</u>-do, <u>must</u>-have aspect of my life." For more on this, see Startup Action 4 (p. **36**).

2. "Doing right eating and living in my healthy-weight range is *easily* doable." For more on weight success mindset, see Startup Action 5 (p. **37**).

ACTION 5: *The night before, do an upcoming-day description with right eating in it.* ✏ Before you go to sleep at night, probably while lying in bed, deliver an upcoming-day description to your subconscious mind. That is, describe to your subconscious mind how you want the next day to turn out. To illustrate, here's some sample wording.

Subconscious mind, tomorrow is going to be a <u>perfect</u> right-eating day. It will happen like this. I will consume my daily calorie allotment of _____ calories for the day, and no more. I'll find this to be <u>easy</u> to do. Each of my daily meals will make me feel like I'm <u>filled up</u>. I will have the full-stomach feeling after each one. And after each one I'll feel <u>fully satisfied</u> for the next _____ hours. And I'll be free of cravings and hunger pangs between meals. It will be a <u>great</u> right-eating day. It will be easy and fun to do, and I'll enjoy it immensely. Subconscious mind, please do whatever you can to positively assist me in making the day happen this way, and in making it be a pleasant, positive day. I believe 100% that you will do this. Thank you very, very much.

Note: This is sample wording, not a must-follow script. Use whatever wording best describes the way you want the day to turn out. And, if you have a nickname for your subconscious mind, you can use that name instead of the name "Subconscious Mind," if you so desire.

Also, if you like, you can repeat this description on the morning of that day. Doing it immediately after waking up, while still lying in bed, is a good time. For more on upcoming-day descriptions, go to "Motivator 3: Upcoming-day Description" (p. **112**) in the Six More Mind Motivators chapter.

ACTION 6: *Reiterate a right-eating backup depiction statement throughout the day.* ✎ Say the following backup depiction statement at least 25 times throughout the day.

I am right now in a right-eating day —
a right-eating day in every single way.

Note: Saying it "at least 25 times" defines a minimum, not a maximum. For extra impact, if you so desire, say it more than 25 times — like say it 40, 50, or even 100 times during the day. For other backup depiction statements you might find helpful in creating right eating, go to "Motivator 2: Backup Depiction Statements" (p. **110**) in the Six More Mind Motivators chapter.

ACTION 7: *Do during-eating self-talk throughout each eating session.* ✎ For how-to instructions, see the During-eating Self-talk section (p. **59**) in Daily Action 5.

OPTIONAL ACTION 8: *Ask God to disclose to you an insight, tactic, or opportunity you might use for ending creeping weight gain.* ✎ My experience has been that when I've requested insight from God on how I might solve a certain problem (of any

kind) or accomplish a certain life-enhancing goal (of any kind), and I've requested it a certain way, I've received what I requested. If you'd like information on that process, go to the *Three Steps to Getting and Using Input from God* section (p. **117**).

Concluding Thoughts

Setback reversal involves a choice between two "stones." Every adversity — challenge, misstep, progress lapse, discouragement — can be viewed either as a millstone pulling you down to failure or as a stepping stone that can lift you to further success. When you view the adversity as a millstone, that's what it becomes. When you view it as a stepping stone, that's what it becomes. So, adopt the Stepping Stone viewpoint for every adversity.

Also, keep in mind that the dividing line between winning and losing is a certain act: the act of converting setbacks into progress actions. So, convert each weight management setback into a progress action and you'll keep lost weight from returning and be a Weight Success Winner for life.

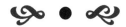

The Weight Success Secret is:
To succeed at healthy-weight living,
do Weight Success Actions every day.
— WHICH MEANS —
The way to overcome an extra-large weight management adversity (challenge, misstep, progress lapse) is:
INCREASE the number, type, duration, and/or intensity of Weight Success Actions you do each day.
~ For more on this subject, see Ch. 14 (p. 116) and Ch. 21 (p. 152) ~

CHAPTER 11: Author's Approach to Eating

This is an example of one person's self-designed dietary approach; it's not provided as a recommended universal program.

IN CASE YOU might find it handy to know, I'm now going to describe my personal approach to eating. But before doing this I must define a term and mention three points.

Definition. A key term used in the Weight Success Method is "preferred dietary program." I define *preferred dietary program* as a set of eating guidelines and eating practices I prefer to follow and which, when followed, cause me to realize good health and healthy-weight living. Another term I use is "preferred eating strategy." It's synonymous with preferred dietary program. Now to three points.

Point One. I'm not saying my eating strategy is the best program or approach for everyone. In my view there's no such thing as "one best dietary program for all."

Point Two. I'm not suggesting that because I use a self-designed program you should too. There are a number of established dietary programs on the market. So there's a good chance at least one of these programs would be a good fit for you.

Point Three. Whatever dietary program or strategy you might choose to go with — and regardless of whether it's a self-designed program or an established program — I suggest you do the five Daily Actions of the Weight Success Method at the same time.

Three Ways Eating Affects Me

Eating impacts my life three ways. Firstly, it affects my *weight*. That is, it either promotes me living at my desired weight <u>or</u> promotes me living at an undesired weight, or overweight. Secondly, it affects my *health*. That is, it either promotes a healthy body <u>or</u> promotes a non-healthy body. Thirdly, it affects the type of daily *pleasure* I experience. That is, I either derive pleasure from right eating <u>or</u> derive it from wrong eating.

So, my eating can impact my life either positively or negatively. The three negative effects are living overweight, poor health, and lack of right-eating pleasure. The three positive effects are living at my desired weight, good health, and experiencing right-eating pleasure. So, what are the factors that determine each of these effects?

Weight Effect. The weight effect derives mainly from the *amount* of food I eat. Meaning, when I eat the right amount of food it moves me toward living in my healthy-weight range. Conversely, when I eat too much food — or frequently engage in overeating — it moves me toward living outside my healthy-weight range, or being overweight.

Health Effect. The health effect derives mainly from the *types* of food I eat. Meaning, when I mostly eat right types of food in proper amounts it promotes me having a healthy body. Conversely, when I mostly eat wrong types of food in certain amounts it promotes me having a non-healthy body.

Pleasure Effect. The pleasure effect depends mainly on the *way* I prepare and eat foods. It also depends on what I *condition* my mind to like. When I prepare and eat foods the right way, and condition myself to like it, I experience right-eating pleasure, which promotes healthy eating. Conversely, when I don't do this I experience wrong-eating pleasure, which promotes non-healthy eating.

So, to sum up: I derive optimal weight, health, and pleasure from my eating by motivating myself to eat right foods in right amounts and by eating in a way that creates right eating enjoyment. Or, put another way, I derive optimal weight, health, and pleasure from applying right eating. The rest of this chapter describes how I do that. For easy identification I call this program the "John Correll Good Health Program."

My Three Eating Objectives

In light of the three ways eating affects me I have three objectives for eating.

Objective one is: Consume an amount of daily calories that results in me living in my healthy-weight range.

Objective two — which goes hand-in-hand with objective one — is: Maintain an optimally healthy body, or maximize the likelihood of living free of debilitating accidents, illnesses, diseases, and bodily malfunction.

Objective three is: Derive maximal pleasure from right eating and minimal pleasure from wrong eating.

Put another way, I strive to enact the three priorities of right eating, as described on page **39** in Startup Action 6.

My Five Guiding Principles

In pursuing these three eating objectives I apply these five principles to my eating.

PRINCIPLE 1: *Whole Mind Involvement.* ✀ Here is a central principle of my approach to eating: My mind — including my subconscious mind — will create the types of thoughts and feelings that guide me toward right eating and away from wrong eating *provided that* (a) I focus each day on right eating and healthy-weight living, (b) I daily communicate to my subconscious mind that I want it to be steering me toward right eating, (c) I hold the belief that it's in the process of doing it, and (d) I express appreciation when right things happen. In briefest form the principle is this: My mind will steer me toward enjoyably living in my healthy-weight range *if* each day I motivate it to do so.

I discovered several years ago that the easiest, most effective way to apply this principle is do the five daily actions of the Weight Success Method (described in Chapter 2). So, this method is the backbone of my eating strategy. Meaning, it's the vehicle by which I get myself to easily, enjoyably

engage in right eating and refrain from wrong eating, or overeating, most of the time.

There are many approaches to enacting weight control. But my experience has led me to conclude that the Weight Success Method is the easiest, cheapest, safest, healthiest, most enjoyable one.

PRINCIPLE 2: *Maximize Pleasure While Minimizing Calories.* ✀ The second principle I apply to eating is this: Each day I strive to maximize the eating pleasure I derive from consuming my daily calorie allotment. My "daily calorie allotment" is the amount of daily calories that results in me living in my healthy-weight range. I've dubbed this principle the "secret to easier calorie control."

I discovered that when I derive only a minimal amount of eating pleasure from my daily calorie allotment I experience "eating-pleasure deprivation," which, in turn, tends to push me toward eating more than I should be eating. But, on the other hand, when I derive a maximal amount of eating pleasure from my daily calorie allotment I experience little or no eating-pleasure deprivation, which, in turn, makes it easier for me to eat a proper amount, or to avoid overeating.

Finally, I discovered that I could maximize the eating pleasure of my daily calorie allotment by applying eight basic eating actions. The *Eight Actions for Easier Calorie Control* chapter (p. **102**) describes these actions. Applying them on a daily basis is part of my approach to eating.

PRINCIPLE 3: *Moderation and Balance.* ✀ The third principle I apply to eating is this. Almost any "bad" food can be eaten without incurring weight gain or ill health *if* it's not eaten to excess. Conversely, almost any "good" food will incur a bad consequence *if* it's eaten to excess. So, achieving good health and weight control is not so much a matter of "always eat this and never eat that" but, rather, is a matter of *moderation and balance.*

So, I diligently strive to eat "good" foods in a healthful amount and refrain from eating "bad" foods to excess. And, as long as I'm doing this — that is, eating "good" foods in a healthful amount and refraining from eating "bad" foods to excess — I don't become angry or upset, or engage in self-criticism, after those occasional times when I happen to eat a small amount of a "bad" food.

PRINCIPLE 4: *Law of Predominant Activity.* ❧ The fourth principle I apply to eating is: When it comes to good health and weight control, what I do only now and then seldom makes a difference but, rather, what makes the difference is what I do *most of the time*. So, I don't hold the goal of "never ever do wrong eating" or "always and forever do right eating." Rather, my objective is to have right eating be my predominant type of eating. So, when now and then I might accidentally or deliberately happen to engage in a small amount of "wrong" eating I don't get angry or upset with myself, or engage in self-criticism.

PRINCIPLE 5: *Twelve-hour Non-eating Period Each Day.* ❧ The fifth principle I apply is: For most days I have a minimum 12-hour non-eating, or "fasting," period each 24-hour day. I do this by avoiding consuming food and beverage, other than water, between 7 p.m. and 7 a.m. In other words, I don't eat between supper and breakfast. Typically, I finish supper by 7 p.m. and start breakfast after 7 a.m.

To conclude, I discovered that applying these five principles makes weight management and eating control easier and more enjoyable.

The Times I Eat

Some research suggests that *when* we eat makes a difference. I suspect this might be true. Although I don't know if there's one universal eating schedule that's best for everyone. So here's the approach that has turned out best for *me*.

Years ago I would do after-dinner, or late-night, snacking. I no longer do that, as indicated by the above Principle 5. After-dinner eating produces unwanted outcomes for me, including weight gain. So, most days my daily eating occurs in the 12-hour period of 7:00 a.m. to 7:00 p.m.

Breakfast. I usually eat breakfast shortly after my daily morning weighing (Daily Action 1). So I do it around 7 or 8 a.m. It's typically a light meal consisting of oatmeal, tomato juice, and perhaps a

small amount of fruit or a small bowl of cold cereal. Total calorie load amounts to around 400–500 calories.

Supper. I usually eat supper around 6 to 7 p.m. It can consist of about anything. But, much of the time it fits the general guidelines and eating practices described in the upcoming two sections. I have no set calorie target for supper. Instead, I use this meal as my *daily calorie adjuster*. It's when I ensure that I consume an amount of daily calories that will keep me in my healthy-weight range. It works like this.

If during-day calorie consumption has been less than usual <u>or</u> if during-day calorie expenditure has been greater than usual — like if I happened to take, say, a long bike ride — my supper meal would likely be slightly larger than usual. Conversely, if during-day calorie consumption has been greater than usual <u>or</u> during-day calorie expenditure has been minimal — like writing all day and doing no exercise — my supper meal would likely be slightly smaller than usual. So, for me, supper is the *pivotal* meal. It's when I ensure that my calorie intake for each day is an amount that will maintain me in my healthy-weight range. Or, put another way, it's when I ensure that each day turns out to be a right-eating day. Which means, supper for me is the "make it or break it time."

Lunch. So, when do I eat lunch? Answer: Any time I get the urge to do it. Meaning, I have no set time for lunch. I might eat it at 10:30 or at noon or at 2:00. I eat it when I'm feeling "hungry for lunch."

<u>Or</u>, I might eat no lunch and, instead, end up just doing a series of mini-snacks through the day, if that's what I feel like. I've found that, for me, sometimes it's easier to subvert hunger pangs and overeating by eating three, four, or five small meals — a.k.a. mini-snacks — throughout the day, or a mini-snack every couple hours, in place of eating one big lunch meal at noon.

Now, in mentioning this mini-snack approach I must impart a warning. Mini-snacking can be a slippery slope. It can easily, unknowingly transform into automatic eating that leads to *over*-snacking that results in excessive daily calorie consumption and weight gain. I speak from personal experience. The reason is, when doing mini-snacking it's easy to overlook doing Daily Action 5 — the guided eating process. So, if you should decide to test out this mini-snack approach, make sure you're doing the guided eating process (p. **56**) *every* time you're doing a mini-snack, no matter how small.

Lastly, I remind you that in describing my approach to eating I'm not suggesting that I think it's the best approach for you. The approach that works for me might or might not work for you. Only you can determine — by personal testing and perhaps physician advice — which eating approach or dietary strategy is best for you.

My Two General Eating Guidelines

Now we come to the question "What types of foods do I focus on eating?" Something that has bugged me for years is the confusing mish-mash of contradictory diets and dietary recommendations. In an attempt to escape this swamp I gravitate to those eating guidelines that have received either governmental endorsement or endorsement of a recognized professional association, such as, for example, the American Heart Association or American Medical Association.

For simplicity, or perhaps sanity, I've distilled this stuff into two eating guidelines. These two guidelines, in conjunction with Principles 1–5, are what I bear in mind when making food decisions.

Eating Guideline 1 – I strive to minimize excessive consumption of:
- high-sugar foods, which includes high-sugar beverages
- refined grains and foods made therefrom
- *trans* fat
- saturated fat
- nitrates and nitrites (i.e., cured or processed meats)
- red meat, especially fatty red meat
- fried foods.

Eating Guideline 2 – I strive to consume an ample, or government-recommended, amount of:
- fruits
- vegetables
- whole grain products
- low-fat and no-fat dairy products
- and occasionally include fish, nuts, and beans (meaning, legumes).

My Specific Eating Practices

Now we come to the specific eating practices I frequently apply. When I put the five principles and two guidelines together, and then translate it into specific actions, what has resulted is the following set of eating practices.

> But here's an important side note. My eating practices are <u>not fixed</u>. Instead, they evolve over time. Meaning, I modify, delete, and add actions as I see fit, for the purpose of producing optimal healthy-weight results and eating enjoyment. I also might modify them as government recommended eating guidelines evolve.

In year 2016, my eating practices generally included the following:

- I drink fat-free milk instead of whole milk most of the time.

- I eat fat-free or low-fat cheese instead of regular or "full-fat" cheese most of the time.

- I eat whole wheat bread instead of white bread much of the time.

- I use reduced-fat butter-type spread instead of regular butter much of the time.

- When I'm using or consuming oil I opt for olive oil most of the time, and when olive oil isn't available I tend to go with canola oil. I minimize solid or hydrogenated fats when I can.

- I opt for low-fat or fat-free salad dressing over regular or "full-fat" dressing most of the time. *Or,* I go with a "half-portion," or reduced amount, of regular dressing and "fortify" its flavor with a sprinkling of red wine vinegar or balsamic vinegar. Tastes great, by the way.

- I use stevia for my main sweetener in place of conventional sugar most of the time. Over the years I've tested a number of non-sugar sweeteners, and finally landed with stevia. For the first week or two of using stevia it seemed to have a "slightly different" sweet flavor to me. But after a couple weeks I ceased noticing the difference, with the result being that stevia and sugar now taste the same to me.

- I eat a bowl of oatmeal cereal almost every morning for breakfast. I go with traditional or "old-fashioned" oatmeal over the quick-cook or instant variety. I eat it with skim milk and add stevia for sweetener. Having oatmeal every morning is easy for me as I like cereal. I've been eating the traditional brands of whole-grain hot and cold cereals since I was about five. Occasionally, along with the oatmeal I include whole wheat toast or a small bowl of whole-grain cold cereal with skim milk and stevia.

- Along with oatmeal for breakfast I drink a small — approximately 5 ounce — glass of tomato juice. I opt for tomato juice over other juices — such as orange, apple, and grape juice — because tomato juice is relatively low in sugar and also lower in calories. I "spike" it with white vinegar in a ratio of 10:1 tomato juice to vinegar. It makes a zippy drink. Plus according to some research, high-acid food tends to diminish the blood glucose spike that can come from eating a glucose-creating food, such as a bowl of oatmeal.

- I drink a glass of water — about 6–8 ounces — with most meals. I'm one of those persons who actually enjoys water and opts for it over most other beverages. Plus I've read that drinking an ample amount of water can produce benefits, such as, for example, reducing the chance of kidney stones.

- I eat fresh fruit almost every day. My home usually has at least three or four kinds in stock at any given time. What I have depends on availability and quality. Typical fruits that can be found in my house include: bananas, apples, pears, peaches, grapes, strawberries, blueberries, raspberries, blackberries, cherries, oranges, tangerines, grapefruit, and melon.

- Supper almost always includes a tossed, or garden, salad and at least one vegetable or vegetable-based ingredient. It also usually includes a starch item, either potato, rice, or pasta. The potato is almost always a baked or roasted version, as opposed to fried. I realize some people frown on eating starchy items, but I eat them for supper. They are, however, prepared with healthy-style cooking methods, which typically means without deep-frying or sautéing.

- I eat reduced-fat or low-fat peanut butter instead of regular or "full-fat" peanut butter. Yup, I do enjoy a peanut butter and jelly sandwich. For that I typically use a reduced-sugar grape or strawberry jelly. Presently, my favorite reduced-fat peanut butter brands are Natural Jif, Reduced-fat Jif, and Smart Balance. All three have great peanut flavor. They, by the way, have nearly identical ingredients. Also, I find that Welch's brand reduced-sugar jellies and spreads suit my taste.

- I use Miracle Whip Light, or reduced fat, in place of regular Miracle Whip for many of my meat, cheese, and tuna fish sandwiches. I also often use mustard as my spread in sandwiches.

- I use low-fat, nitrate/nitrite-free deli sliced turkey for most of my meat sandwiches.

- For making hamburgers, chili, tacos, and the like I go with low-fat ground beef — that is, ground beef made to contain no more than about 4–6 percent fat. And, in most of my home cooking I tend to avoid "regular" ground beef or hamburger, which typically has a fat content of 20 percent or more.

- I often include a can of "light" or "heart healthy" soup for lunch. I typically go with something like vegetable beef or chicken noodle or chicken rice or Manhattan-style seafood chowder, for examples. Light-style soups typically contain two servings per can and have a per-serving calorie load in the 80–110 range, or 160–220 calories per can. Sometimes when I'm extra hungry I'll "fortify" the soup with some canned vegetables or leftover vegetables from the prior night's dinner. Or, in the case of seafood chowder I might add a small (3 oz) can of tuna fish, or in the case of chicken soup a small (3 oz) can of chicken.

- When I get a hankering for a cookie I typically eat a low-fat graham cracker or perhaps a few animal crackers. Believe it or not, animal crackers are one of my favorite cookies. Plus they're relatively low in fat and sugar, as cookies go. I like the Stauffer's brand best, but find the Nabisco version to be good, too.

- For home-stocked ice cream I gravitate toward the fat-free and reduced-fat versions. To me, Breyers fat-free ice cream—chocolate, vanilla, or strawberry—and also Edy's "1/2 the fat" ice cream have decent flavor and texture. I usually eat my ice cream in a cake cone rather than in a dish, thereby prolonging eating pleasure.

- Sometimes I have popcorn. I go with the low-fat varieties, which have about 100–120 calories per serving. This is a great way to satisfy a salty-snack hankering with relatively few calories and very little "harmful" ingredient. I eat it one kernel at a time, thereby prolonging eating pleasure.

- Occasionally I have a fried egg sandwich. Actually, it's not a true fried egg as I use no fat but, instead, I "fry" it with a non-stick skillet, with little or no fat added. I put the fried egg on top of a piece of unbuttered low-cal whole wheat toast and add a slice of fat-free or low-fat cheese on top of the egg. When the slice of cheese is applied while the egg is still hot the cheese slightly melts over the egg. The result is a tasty open-faced egg sandwich. Sometimes for variety I'll grill up a couple slices of low-fat soy-

protein "bacon," which my family lovingly calls "fakin' bacon," and add that on top of the cheese. And, when I feel like going all-out I include a couple slices of tomato between the bread and egg. This results in a nutritious, tasty, low fat egg-bacon-tomato-cheese sandwich.

- While I can't say I eat soy-protein foods extensively, I do enjoy them now and then. Two items stocked in my freezer are soy-protein Bacon Strips (mentioned above) and soy-protein Black Bean Burger, both made by Morning Star Farms. According to the manufacturer, the Bacon Strips have 44 percent less fat than regular pork bacon and the Black Bean Burger has 73 percent less fat than regular ground beef.

  When heated in a skillet, as opposed to a microwave, both products are tasty and satisfying. The bean burger is especially good when topped with a dab of thousand island dressing plus the usual burger condiments of dill pickle, cheese, and sliced tomato. Lastly, please know that I mention the Morning Star Farms name as a point of reference and not to imply that it's the only maker of good soy-protein-based foods.

- To obtain the right amount of daily fiber I go with whole psyllium husk as a supplement. I prefer it over other fiber sources because it provides both types of fiber: soluble and insoluble — in a ratio of about 75% soluble, 25% insoluble. I purchase it in bulk form — large can, bottle, or bag — from a health food store or a well-stocked supermarket. Psyllium husk, by the way, happens to be the main fiber-providing ingredient in Metamucil.

  I include the psyllium husk with my breakfast and supper meals. At breakfast I add a *rounded* tablespoon to my bowl of oatmeal. This provides about four grams of added fiber. But, if I deem it to be desirable I'll increase the portion slightly. For supper I combine the same amount into a small portion of cold cereal, usually

Grape-nuts Flakes, and eat it as a "dessert" after supper. Or, in place of that, I might sprinkle it over a tossed salad, after the dressing has been added. Or, I might stir the psyllium into a large glass of water and drink it right before starting eating. Note: Psyllium husk is nearly taste-free, so it leaves the flavor of whatever it's added to — like a salad or bowl of cereal — virtually unchanged.

At supper I might adjust the psyllium portion amount based on what I figure my fiber intake has been for that day. If it seems like I've consumed an above-average amount of fiber, via the foods I've eaten, I reduce the psyllium portion slightly at suppertime. Conversely, if I figure I consumed a below-average amount of fiber in that day I increase the psyllium portion slightly.

Clarifying Comments

In the above description I use the word "I" extensively, as in "I prepare" this and "I stock" that. This conveys an impression that I'm a one-man dietary dynamo doing everything myself. In actuality, my wife and life partner Janet does most of our food shopping, which happens to be her preference, and also prepares most of our at-home supper meals, which is her preference.

This conveys the impression that I do nothing regarding dietary decision-making, food shopping, and kitchen duties. But that's not the case, either. I make trips to the market for certain foods, and will convey to Janet, via our weekly shopping list, requests for specific foods. Fortunately for me, she's accommodating of my food-related requests and suggestions, and even sometimes takes the initiative to buy or prepare something new that she thinks I might like to "test out."

Also, by the way, as regards suppertime kitchen duties Janet and I take a team approach. She does meal preparation; I do after-meal clean-up. It typically requires 30 to 60 minutes on her part to prepare a supper, and 20 to 30 minutes on my part for clean-up. So I figure I'm getting a good deal.

I now reiterate a point made at the opening of this chapter. Which is: By relating my personal approach to eating I am *not* suggesting that it's necessarily the most productive approach for you. And, just because I happen to apply a self-designed dietary program, as opposed to one of the established programs, I am *not* saying that a self-designed eating program is the best way to go for you. In fact, I happen to believe that for many persons an established dietary program is the easiest, most effective, most rewarding way to do dieting, or dietary management.

But regardless of what dietary program or strategy you apply — and regardless of whether you go the design-it-yourself route or the established program route — there's an additional thing you should do. Along with doing your preferred dietary program *also* do the five daily actions of the Weight Success Method at the same time. Doing this likely will make the dietary program of your choice easier and more effective.

What Should Be the Rule?

When it comes to good health and weight control, what you do only now and then seldom makes a difference. Rather, what usually makes the big difference is what you do most of the time. So, unless it's something you can absolutely attain, it might be best to forego absolute-type rules like "never engage in overeating" or "always and forever do non-overeating."

Instead, a more productive approach might be to have non-overeating be your main type of eating, as opposed to being your only type of eating. So when now and then you accidentally or deliberately happen to engage in a small amount of overeating, there's no need to feel angry, guilty, discouraged, sinful, weak, or any other counterproductive negative emotion. In short, the question is this.

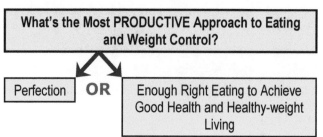

What's Your #1 Eating Goal?

For most persons their #1 eating goal is maximize pleasure. But this leads to overeating and weight gain. So, I suggest you make your #1 eating goal to be: maintain body weight in your healthy-weight range. Then, within that context, make goal #2 to be: promote good health, and goal #3 to be: gain maximal eating pleasure from right eating — in that order of priority. When you do this you'll find that creating healthy-weight living becomes much **EASIER.**

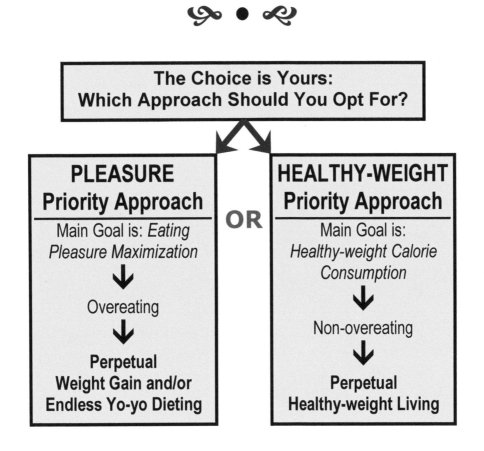

The Choice is Yours:
Which Approach Should You Opt For?

PLEASURE
Priority Approach

Main Goal is: *Eating Pleasure Maximization*

↓

Overeating

↓

Perpetual Weight Gain and/or Endless Yo-yo Dieting

OR

HEALTHY-WEIGHT
Priority Approach

Main Goal is: *Healthy-weight Calorie Consumption*

↓

Non-overeating

↓

Perpetual Healthy-weight Living

CHAPTER 12: Eight Actions for Easier Calorie Control

Calorie control can be easier and more enjoyable than you likely imagine,
if you go about it the right way.

IF YOU DESIRE to maximize eating pleasure while also controlling calorie intake, apply the eight simple actions in this chapter. These actions pertain to my second eating principle: maximize pleasure while minimizing calories (p. **95**).

When it comes to calorie control most people hold an erroneous belief. They believe controlling calorie intake is hard to do. So, they hate pursuing any dietary program that involves calorie control, which many programs do. Truth is, controlling daily calorie intake is easier and more enjoyable with a certain approach. This chapter describes that approach. But before disclosing it I must lay some groundwork.

The Dilemma in Eating

Most of us eat to satisfy two objectives: (1) to acquire nourishment and energy and (2) to derive eating pleasure. But while deriving eating pleasure a nasty side-effect usually crops up: *weight gain*. Weight gain comes from consuming more calories than our body is metabolizing, or "burning up." We call this overeating. Initially this weight gain is merely a nuisance. Eventually, however, it grows into a problem. When this happens some persons adopt a third objective: *weight control*.

Most weight-control programs involve one or both of two strategies. The first strategy is to enact a higher level of physical activity, called exercise. This results in burning up the "extra calories" we're consuming.

The second strategy is to consume an amount of daily calories that's equal to the amount of calories our body has been burning up. This involves daily calorie control.

Many persons find using both strategies in combination produces the quickest results. But you need to know that the first strategy — exercise — is optional, while the second strategy — calorie control — is must-do. Why? Because it's possible for most folks to achieve and maintain their desired healthy weight without exercise. But, except for those engaged in very high levels of physical activity, most of us cannot achieve and maintain our desired weight without controlling calorie intake. So, contrary to what many people assume, calorie control is a vital requirement for weight management success, and exercise is not. Which, of course, is not to say you should forget about exercise.

Unfortunately, when most of us attempt to enact calorie control a problem arises. In our effort to reduce calories we end up consuming less food. In consuming less food we derive less eating pleasure. This reduction in eating pleasure creates a feeling of pleasure deprivation, or withdrawal. Finally, this feeling of pleasure deprivation drives us back to eating the types and the amount of food we previously derived pleasure from. The result: We fail at calorie control and, thereby, fail at weight control.

What makes calorie control so tricky is it involves a dilemma. It happens to be a universal dilemma of dieters. That dilemma is this. When we consume an amount of calories that results in putting or keeping our body weight in our desired weight range we end up with a reduced amount of eating pleasure and also nagging hunger pangs much of the time. On the other hand, when we consume the amount of food that gives us maximum eating pleasure and a feeling of fullness we end up overeating and acquiring fat.

So, the dilemma comes down to this. Should I live with a reduced calorie intake, which results in eating pleasure deprivation *or* should I live with a non-reduced calorie intake, which results in endless overeating and fat gain? Each is a bad option.

Most people assume there's no way out of this dilemma. But there is a way. It involves a third option: Adopt a two-prong eating strategy of maximizing eating pleasure while controlling calorie intake. Applying this strategy involves a certain perspective. So I'm now going to describe that perspective. After that comes the "secret to easier calorie control."

Best Perspective for Controlling Calories

For maximal effectiveness, approach calorie control like this. Pretend that when you arise each morning you're given a bag of calories to use for that day. This bag of calories is your *healthy-weight calorie allotment*. It's the maximum number of calories you can consume each day and still achieve or maintain your desired healthy weight. Each day you may use all the allotted calories or only part of them. But you absolutely are not allowed to consume more calories than are in your "healthy-weight calorie allotment bag." Lastly, it's up to you and your qualified health advisor to determine how many calories your healthy-weight calorie allotment should consist of.

What's more, pretend that you have an eating mission. Assume that this mission is to derive maximum eating pleasure from the bag of calories you've been allotted for each day. To succeed at this mission you must treat your allotment of daily calories like precious currency. That is, you must spend it wisely. You must spend it in a way that maximizes your eating pleasure.

When you do this you avoid, or at least greatly reduce, eating pleasure deprivation. This, in turn, makes it easier for you to control your calorie intake and stick with your preferred dietary program; thus, making it easier for you to create healthy-weight living.

So, how do you accomplish your eating mission? You apply seven eating actions. I call them *pleasure-maximizing eating actions*. By applying these seven actions you maximize the eating pleasure from your healthy-weight calorie allotment and, thereby, make calorie control non-painful and easier.

So, in a nutshell the secret to easier calorie control is: *Each day maximize the eating pleasure of your healthy-weight calorie allotment*. Now,

here in summary form are seven actions for doing that.

1. Dispense with low-pleasure, high-calorie add-ons.
2. Reduce the portion amount of high-pleasure, high-calorie add-ons.
3. Replace high-calorie foods with lower-calorie foods that still yield eating pleasure.
4. Choose foods that deliver a longer duration of eating pleasure per calorie consumed.
5. Eat in a way that lengthens the duration of eating pleasure per calorie consumed.
6. Season foods in a way that increases the amount of pleasurable palate sensation.
7. Replace high-cal snacks with low-cal and no-cal snacks.

Apply these seven actions on a daily basis. It enables you to each day maximize the eating pleasure of your healthy-weight calorie allotment. Which, in turn, makes for easier calorie control. Also, along with these seven actions include one more action: Action 8. I'll now describe these eight actions, which lead to easier calorie-control success.

ACTION 1: Dispense with low-pleasure, high-calorie add-ons.

Virtually every item you eat provides pleasure. But items differ in the amount of pleasure per calorie that they provide. Some deliver a large amount of pleasure for a small amount of calories. Others deliver a small amount of pleasure for a large amount of calories. Since you have only a certain number of calories to work with — that being your healthy-weight calorie allotment — you should do these two things. Firstly, focus on foods that deliver a greater amount of pleasure per calorie. Secondly, shun foods that deliver a lesser amount of pleasure per calorie, while maintaining a healthy balanced diet, of course. View the situation like this.

Greater pleasure per calorie = *Good Food*

Lesser pleasure per calorie = *Bad Food*

Good Foods create **maximal** pleasure for your healthy-weight calorie allotment

Bad Foods create **minimal** pleasure for your healthy-weight calorie allotment

So, focus on "good foods" — those that deliver greater eating pleasure per calorie. And, shun "bad foods" — those that deliver lesser eating pleasure per calorie.

One of the easiest ways to reduce your consumption of "bad foods" is eliminate add-ons. Indeed, omitting an add-on often turns a "bad food" into a "good food." An *add-on* is something that's added to another food to change its taste or texture. Many of the calories most persons consume come from add-ons. These items tend to be high in fat or, in some cases, consist totally of fat. Examples of high-calorie add-ons include fat-based spreads, such as butter and margarine, and high-fat dressings, sauces, and condiments. For certain food items, add-ons can constitute 20, 30, or even 50 percent or more of the total calorie load of the food. Ditto for an entire meal.

Examples

I'll illustrate. To begin, consider how most persons make a sandwich. First they get a slice of bread. It contains between 50 to 100 calories. Then they apply one to two tablespoons of butter or margarine to the slice. This constitutes 100 to 200 calories. So let's see — original slice of bread equals 100 calories, add-on equals 100 calories, total calories for the modified slice: 200 calories. Wow, is this add-on really needed? Why not just make the sandwich without the 100 to 200 calories of low-pleasure butter spread? The sandwich's taste will be nearly identical to what it is with the add-on. Within a week or two, especially after delivering a mini-directive to your mind, you'll not miss the butter or margarine you once had in your sandwiches.

Here's another example. Consider how most people eat a pancake or waffle or French toast. The first thing they do is slather it with butter or margarine. So, what they end up with is this. Original pancake equals 200 calories, butter equals 200 calories, total calories for the modified pancake: 400 calories. This is crazy. Why not just eat the pancake without the 200 calories of add-on butter spread? Just add a little of your usual sweetener — like some reduced-sugar syrup, or reduced-sugar jam, or sliced fruit, or government-approved artificial sweetener — and enjoy the pancake without the added calories and, by the way, without the added saturated fat. The pancake's taste will be nearly identical to what it is with the butter or margarine. After eating it this way a few times you'll not miss the butter.

A similar thing often happens with eating a roll or a muffin. Many persons apply a thick dollop of butter or margarine to it. Instead, try eating these foods plain, or with nothing on them. You might be surprised. You might discover, as I did, that the bread, roll, or muffin tastes as good without the add-on as with it.

Ditto for potatoes and vegetables. A quality potato or vegetable, properly prepared and with a touch of seasoning, tastes great — every bit as good as one floating in a sea of butter or smothered with sauce, gravy, sour cream, or any of the many other taste-altering, calorie-adding add-ons.

There's a reason why this is so. It's because add-ons don't always enhance the flavor of a food. We just erroneously assume they do. Instead, an add-on often masks a food's original flavor rather than improves it. When you dispense with the add-on you can enjoy the pure taste of the original food. Sometimes the pure taste is even more enjoyable than the masked or altered taste of the modified food. We just never learned to enjoy the original flavor because we've been eating food smothered with add-ons from about age two.

Question

Now here's the key question. In any of these examples, are the 100 to 200 calories of add-on really worth it? If the answer's "no," *dispense with it.*

Another way of framing the question is: Can I get a bigger pleasure bang from my healthy-weight calorie allotment by dispensing with this low-pleasure add-on? Or, in other words: Can I make better use of the 100 or 200 calories consumed by this add-on? By "better use" I mean, using the add-on's calories in a way that produces greater eating pleasure.

If the answer's "yes," dispense with the add-on. Put those saved calories to better use. You have two options. First, use the saved calories for consuming some other food that provides greater pleasure than the low-pleasure add-on. Second, don't use the calories at all. That is, reduce your calorie intake for the day by the amount of calories you saved. Either option enables you to more easily achieve your calorie intake goal.

ACTION 2: Reduce the portion amount of high-pleasure, high-calorie add-ons.

So, what about add-ons that are high calorie but also deliver high pleasure for you? For these items reduce the portion amount. As explained in Action 1, many persons use huge portions of add-ons. They use way more than what's needed to impart the desired flavor. So, for these cut the portion of high-pleasure add-ons by half or more.

You'll discover that a 50 percent reduction in portion amount often results in only about a 10 percent reduction in flavor. In other words, with many add-ons the first 50 percent of the portion amount creates 90 percent of the flavor enhancement. And, the second 50 percent adds little or nothing. As a result, the second 50 percent of the portion amount can be viewed as wasted calories that can be put to better use. So, cut the portion amount of high-pleasure, high-calorie add-ons by half or more. Amazingly, you won't miss this portion of the add-on.

Also, try substituting a portion of the high-calorie add-on with a low-calorie or no-calorie add-on. For example, with salads you can cut the portion amount of dressing in half and then add a squeeze of lemon juice or sprinkle of vinegar to the salad to replace the flavor that's lost from the missing half-portion of dressing. It works great. And, you're consuming only half as many calories in salad dressing. This can greatly reduce the overall calorie load of a salad.

Then, put those saved calories to better use. Either (a) use them to up your eating pleasure by enjoying some other food that delivers greater pleasure or (b) don't use them at all and, thereby, reduce your calorie intake for that day.

ACTION 3: Replace high-calorie foods with lower-calorie foods that still yield eating pleasure.

Much of what I've said about add-ons also applies to an entire food type. Many foods, including beverages, come in high, medium, and low calorie levels. The high level is usually labeled "regular" or "traditional" or "original" or "classic." Medium is often labeled "reduced calorie." And, low is labeled "low-calorie" or "no-calorie" or "calorie-free".

Milk is a good example. You can get it in 3-percent fat (whole milk), 2-percent fat (reduced fat milk), ½-percent fat (low fat milk), and no-fat (skim milk). Many persons turn up their nose at reduced-fat and no-fat milk. But you can use it to reduce calorie intake. Whole milk (3-percent fat) is 145 calories per cup or eight ounces. Skim milk is just 85 calories per cup — nearly 40 percent fewer calories. If you're a milk drinker, as I am, switching from whole milk to skim milk frees up a lot of calories per day that could be put to some other possibly more productive use. It also greatly reduces your saturated fat intake. Check the Nutrition Facts box on the label. The saturated fat difference is eye-opening.

A similar situation applies to many other food products. They come in high-calorie versions, reduced-calorie versions, and low-calorie versions. Examples include beer, ice cream, cheese, bread, salad dressings, spreads, soups, and dessert items or sweet treats. It goes on and on. In many cases the reduced-calorie version — and sometimes even the low-calorie version — carries nearly as much pleasing taste as the high-calorie version.

ACTION 4: Choose foods that deliver a longer duration of eating pleasure per calorie consumed.

Foods vary in duration of eating pleasure they provide. Some provide no more than a few seconds of eating pleasure. Others provide several minutes or more. Plus here's the catch. Oftentimes both foods contain the same amount of calories. So, which food do you want to be eating? The one that delivers 10 seconds of eating pleasure for X amount of calories? *Or*, the one that delivers, say, five minutes of eating pleasure for the same X amount of calories? Obviously, you gain more eating pleasure per calorie with the second one. So, choose that one and avoid the first one.

So evaluate your food choices in terms of calories consumed per minute of eating pleasure. The fewer calories consumed per minute of eating pleasure, the better. Here's the formula for it:

Calorie Load of the Food ÷ Minutes of Eating Time = Calories Per Minute of Eating Pleasure

I call it *Calories Per Minute of Pleasure* formula. I'll illustrate how it works.

EXAMPLE 1: Ice Cream. You can eat ice cream one of two ways: in a bowl or in a cone. In a bowl you consume the ice cream in about one minute. The same amount in a cone takes you three to five minutes. So, you gain two to four extra minutes of eating pleasure with the cone. Here's how it works with the calories per minute of pleasure formula. Let's assume the ice cream portion contains 200 calories and the cone is 10 calories.

Calories Per Minute of Pleasure with the bowl = **200** calories per minute (200 calories ÷ 1 minute)

Calories Per Minute of Pleasure with the cone = **52** calories per minute (210 calories ÷ 4 minutes)

I'll take the cone every time.

EXAMPLE 2: Popsicles. To get three or four minutes of low-calorie eating pleasure have a popsicle. You loved 'em when you were a kid and, guess what, they still taste great. To achieve maximum pleasure bang per calorie, check out the no-sugar-added versions, which are about 15 calories. It's like three minutes of eating pleasure for free!

EXAMPLE 3: Reduced-fat popcorn. A bowl of individual-portion popcorn can take 10 to 15 minutes to eat when eaten one kernel at a time. A typical individual portion of reduced-fat popcorn has about 100 calories. If it takes you 10 minutes to eat, that amounts to just 10 calories per minute of eating pleasure (100 calories divided by 10 minutes). By comparison, if you eat a typical cookie in, say, one minute, that could amount to 100 or more calories per minute of eating pleasure. This is ten times more calories per minute than in eating reduced-fat popcorn.

So, when making food choices use the calories per minute of pleasure formula. It's a nifty way of gaining maximum eating pleasure from your healthy-weight calorie allotment.

ACTION 5: Eat in a way that lengthens the duration of eating pleasure per calorie consumed.

This action goes hand-in-hand with Action 4. In Action 4 you select foods that take longer to eat. In this action you eat foods in a way that results in lengthened eating time. In both cases the goal is the same: to derive more pleasure bang for your daily calorie allotment by lengthening the duration of pleasure-producing eating time.

You can lengthen the duration of eating three ways. First, take smaller bites and smaller swallows. Second, chew slower or longer. Third, pause between bites. For this you might have a sip of water or a little conversation. In short, try to avoid gobbling food and gulping beverage and, instead, savor it.

ACTION 6: Season foods in a way that increases the amount of pleasurable palate sensation.

Seasoning often determines the amount of pleasure you derive from a food. The most common seasoning is salt. After that, black pepper. But other seasoning options abound. Consider the many herbs, spices, hot sauces, condiments, and vinegars. Nearly all are low in calories. Many are calorie-free.

Use these seasonings to increase the pleasure you derive from food. For an example, here's a snack tactic I sometimes use to satisfy a "craving for flavor" without consuming a lot of calories. I get some tomato juice and pour about six ounces into a glass. Then, I stir in some ground black pepper, oregano, hot sauce, a squeeze of lemon, and perhaps a dash of Worcestershire sauce. I use enough of the hot items to create a fiery flavor. Then I enjoy this along with a dill pickle or some other high-flavor, low-calorie snack item. If when I'm done my mouth isn't screaming "Great, great … enough, enough … I'm happy now," it means I probably didn't put enough seasoning and hot sauce into the tomato juice. Next time I experiment with upping the seasoning or hot sauce.

ACTION 7: Replace high-cal snacks with low-cal and no-cal snacks.

Some diet programs tell you to eliminate snacking between meals. For many people this is good advice. But if ending all between-meal snacking results in eating pleasure deprivation, which in turn results in leaving the diet program, then this might be not-so-good advice.

When the latter condition applies, do this Action 7: Switch from high-calorie between-meal snacks to low-calorie or no-calorie snacks. Use these snacks to neutralize a craving or a nagging desire to experience eating pleasure.

Also, combine this Action 7 with Action 5. That is, eat your low-cal snacks in small bites or small sips to maximize the duration of eating pleasure you derive.

•

So to sum up this far, the secret to easier calorie control is: *Each day maximize the eating pleasure of your healthy-weight calorie allotment.* Do it by applying the above Actions 1–7. Plus, also apply this Action 8.

ACTION 8: Know the calorie load of what you're eating (or about to eat).

To achieve easier calorie control, bear in mind the calorie load of the food you're consuming or are thinking of consuming. By doing this it causes your mind to steer you toward correct calorie consumption. It also makes it easier for you to maximize the pleasure of your healthy-weight calorie allotment with Actions 1, 3, 4, and 7. Here are two ways you can know the calorie load of what you eat.

1 – Look at the Nutrition Facts Box

The easiest way to get calorie info is check the **Nutrition Facts** box. It appears on the package of nearly every food item. It will tell you the *calories per portion* and also total calories for the entire container. Make it a habit to check this information and to know the calorie load of what you eat or are thinking of eating.

Also, restaurants are starting to tell us the calorie amount of their menu items. Sometimes it can be found on the menu or on the back of a placemat or in a pamphlet. Many post it on their website.

For the rare food item that comes without printed nutrition info you can usually find this information on the Internet, such as, for example at:

calorieking.com

Also, when making a decision about whether to eat something it can help to know the amount of exercise that would be required to burn up the number of calories consumed by eating it. So, when you see the *calories per serving* number on a menu or in the Nutrition Facts box on a package it sometimes can help to refer to this chart (next page).

Calories Burned Per Hour				
	BODY WEIGHT			
ACTIVITY (1 hr.)	130 lb	155 lb	180 lb	205 lb
Brisk Walking (3.5 mph)	224	267	311	354
Slow Running (5 mph)	472	563	654	745
Mod. Cycling (12–13.9 mph)	472	563	654	745
Weight-lifting, light workout	177	211	245	279

This chart lists four exercise activities. For each of the activities it tells you the number of calories you burn in one hour. So, for example, if you weigh around 155 pounds and do brisk walking for one hour you burn about 267 calories. To extend the example, if you eat something that contains 267 calories and you weigh in the neighborhood of 155 pounds you would have to do one hour of brisk walking to burn the calories in that portion of food. Suggestion: Make a copy of this chart and carry it in your wallet or purse for quick reference. For info on calories burned by other types of activities, go to:

nutristrategy.com

The numbers in this chart come from there.

2 – Use Food-measuring Tools at Home

As with most every pursuit, to excel at it it helps to have the right tools. To excel at calorie control, especially if you do a lot of home cooking, these three food measuring tools can be helpful:

1. Set of measuring spoons and perhaps a set of dry-measure measuring cups;

2. Liquid-measure measuring cup; and

3. Portion scale with at least a sixteen ounce maximum capacity divided into quarter-ounce incre-

ments or smaller — or, in metric, at least a 500 gram maximum capacity divided into five-gram increments or smaller.

TIP: If you're serious about calorie control, a portion scale and measuring cups can be very helpful.

Concluding Summary

The secret to easier calorie control is: *Each day maximize the eating pleasure of your healthy-weight calorie allotment* (Actions 1–7), plus bear in mind the calorie load of what you eat (Action 8). As an infographic it works like this.

Eight Key Calorie-control Activities

1. Dispense with low-pleasure, high-cal add-ons.
2. Reduce the portion amount of high-pleasure, high-calorie add-ons.
3. Replace high-calorie foods with lower-calorie foods that still yield eating pleasure.
4. Choose foods that deliver a longer duration of eating pleasure per calorie consumed.
5. Eat in a way that lengthens the duration of eating pleasure per calorie consumed.
6. Season foods in a way that increases the amount of pleasurable palate sensation.
7. Replace high-cal snacks with low-cal snacks.
8. Know the calorie load of what you're eating.

Creates maximum eating pleasure from your healthy-weight calorie allotment.

Results in you more easily controlling calorie intake and achieving right eating and, ultimately, healthy-weight living — especially when done in conjunction with the Weight Success Method.

Either you control calories or calories control you. The easiest way to gain control over calories is (a) wring maximum pleasure from those you should be eating, then (b) spurn the rest.

What's Your #1 Priority in Eating?

Having *pleasure maximization* as a #1 priority in eating promotes overeating and weight gain. To avoid this, make **healthy-weight calorie consumption** your #1 priority. Then make your #2 and #3 priorities the deriving of optimal health and maximal pleasure from those calories. When you do this you'll find that creating healthy-weight living becomes easier. For more, see the Right Eating section, page **39**, in Startup Action 6.

❧ ● ❧

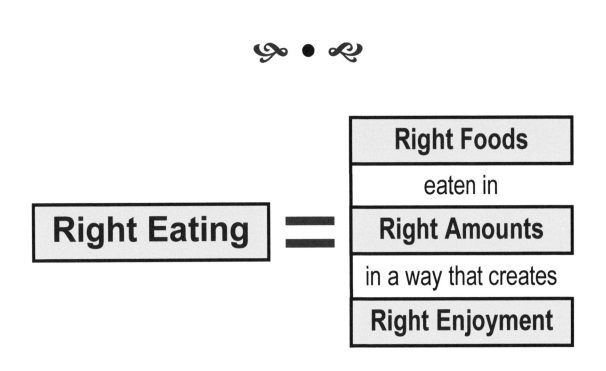

Right Eating **=**

Right Foods
eaten in
Right Amounts
in a way that creates
Right Enjoyment

CHAPTER 13: Six More Mind Motivators

To some people more is better. So here's MORE — six additional, optional, powerful ways to motivate your mind to assist you with creating healthy-weight living.

MOST PEOPLE will find that doing the five daily actions of the Weight Success Method is sufficient to motivate their mind to steer them toward living in their healthy-weight range. But in every pursuit there are those who desire to progress a little faster or gain extra expertise. If you happen to be one of these persons, this chapter is for you. All you need do is apply one or more of these six optional mind motivators. In doing this you might use the test-it-out approach. That is, pick one of the six and try it for a week. If it increases your healthy-weight focus and effectiveness, make that motivator an add-on to the five daily actions of the Weight Success Method. If it doesn't do much for you, drop it and test another one. Here now are six optional mind motivators.

MOTIVATOR 1:
High-frequency Goal Statement

Say your Healthy-weight Goal Statement *more than* 25 times a day.

Daily Action 4 of the Weight Success Method instructs you to say your Healthy-weight Goal Statement at least 25 times each day. Note: "at least 25 times each day" defines a minimum, not a maximum. So if you'd like to increase your mind's focus on realizing healthy-weight living say the Goal Statement more than 25 times a day. Like, say it 40 or 50 or even 100 times a day. As explained in Daily Action 4, you can easily do this by fitting Goal Statement iterations into the "free time" periods of your day, or into those times when you can do Statement iterations while also doing something else at the same time. Regarding that, here's a couple powerful suggestions to try.

Nighttime Iterations

Some persons sleep through an entire night without waking. But many arise at least once to go to the bathroom. If you do that, take advantage of it.

Silently deliver either your Healthy-weight Goal Statement or a backup depiction statement after you come back to bed. (Upcoming Motivator 2 lists backup depiction statements.) Do this by repeating the statement in your mind as you're falling asleep. Delivering healthy-weight messages at this time can produce powerful results.

Waking-up Iterations

When you awaken in the morning, and while still lying in bed with your eyes closed and mind relaxed, say your Healthy-weight Goal Statement three times in your mind. Or, for extra effect, say it ten times, which takes only about 40 to 50 seconds.

Saying your Healthy-weight Goal Statement at these two times — when you awaken at night and first thing in the morning while waking up — can produce a powerful effect.

Plus, in addition to increasing the number of times you say your Healthy-weight Goal Statement also increase your emotional intensity when saying it. You need not do this for all iterations but it could be worthwhile to do it for at least a few.

MOTIVATOR 2:
Backup Depiction Statements

Say a backup depiction statement at least 10 times a day.

Your Healthy-weight Goal Statement (in Daily Action 4) is a form of verbal depiction. A verbal depiction is a word description of a situation. Typically the situation being depicted is either (a) an imagined desired situation you want to actualize, or make real or (b) a desirable present situation you want to perpetuate, such as continuing to live in your healthy-weight range.

Your Healthy-weight Goal Statement is the primary verbal depiction used — or daily iterated — in the Weight Success Method. It produces great results. But by including iterations of a backup depiction statement each day you can *increase* results. Coming up in the next column is a list of backup statements you can use for this.

How Backup Statements Work. Backup depiction statements work with your Healthy-weight Goal Statement to expedite healthy-weight living. Your Goal Statement portrays your ultimate goal. Which is, to live your life as a person of your healthy weight. Each of the backup depiction statements describes a means or situation for helping bring about this ultimate goal. When a backup depiction statement is said on the same day as your Healthy-weight Goal Statement it causes your mind to focus on both your ultimate goal and a means for getting it. This can be powerful.

What to Do. Pick a backup depiction statement that looks interesting, or that appears like it might help fix a certain problem or achieve a certain goal. For example, if you're having trouble with over-snacking you might find backup depiction statement #5 (in the list coming up) to be effective, or if you're eating too much at meals you might use statement #6.

Then use the chosen statement for a week. *Say it at least 10 times each day.* Do this along with saying your Healthy-weight Goal Statement, not in place of it. If it produces desired results, keep using it. If it doesn't, drop it and test another one. Note: It's okay to use two or more depiction statements the same day. Also bear in mind, the power of depiction statements derives from repetition. The more repetition, the greater the power. Here are 11 sample statements to choose from.

11 Optional Backup Depiction Statements

1. *I am right now in a guided-eating week. I do guided eating every time I eat.*
   (Note: Guided eating is described in Daily Action 5 of the Weight Success Method, page 56.)

2. *I am right now in a right-eating day — a right-eating day in every single way.*

3. *I am right now in a right-eating day — less than _____ calories is what I eat today.*
   (In the blank space, insert a number of calories.)

4. *I am right now forever <u>free</u> of every wrong-eating habit that's ever been with me.*

5. *I am right now forever <u>free</u> of the over-snacking habit that used to be with me.*

6. *I am right now forever <u>free</u> of the mealtime gluttony-eating that once appealed to me.*

7. *Healthy weight, BENEFITS — Overweight, PAIN. <u>Steer</u> me to the benefits — <u>Save</u> me from the pain.*

8. *I control eating — eating doesn't control me.*

9. *I'm living each day in my healthy-weight range.*

10. *I focus each day on healthy-weight living.*

11. *I weigh _____, _____, _____.*
    (In each of the three blank spaces, insert your ideal weight number.)

Optional Wording. Feel free to modify any statement to best fit your situation. For example, in statements 2 and 3 you can replace the word "right-eating" with "healthy-eating," if you wish. Also, in statement 4 you can replace "wrong-eating" with "overeating." And, in statements #4 and #5 you can replace "habit" with "urge."

Make Your Own. Also, reading the above statements might give you ideas for backup depiction statements of your own creation. If so, write them up and test them. Tip: The "listening audience" for depiction statements is your mind — in particular your subconscious mind. Remember this when crafting the wording for your statements.

Definition of Key Terms Used in the Depiction Statements

Right-eating day (a.k.a. healthy-eating day): A day in which your overall eating for the day amounts to right eating (a.k.a. healthy-weight eating).

Wrong eating (a.k.a. non-healthy eating): Eating that hinders good health or hinders living in your healthy-weight range.

Over-snacking: Eating too much or too many times between meals, resulting in overeating for the day.

Mealtime gluttony-eating: Eating until stuffed, or until your stomach can hold no more; or overeating during meals.

Healthy-weight living (a.k.a. right-weight living): Living in your healthy-weight range.

MOTIVATOR 3:
Upcoming-day Description

In the morning right after waking, tell your mind how you want the upcoming day to happen.

Many people often lie in bed for a few minutes in the morning after waking up. If you happen to be one who does this you can use that time for powerful results.

While lying in bed, with your eyes closed and mind relaxed, sometimes called resting-mind mode, silently — in your mind — say your Healthy-weight Goal Statement three times.

Then, with your eyes still closed, communicate to your mind — or, more specifically, to your subconscious mind — how you want the upcoming day to turn out, especially as pertains to eating. Tell it *exactly* what you want it to help make happen.

So, what do you describe? To answer this question consider the following.

Would you like to go through the day without being harassed by the over-snacking habit or by the mealtime gluttony-eating habit or by unwanted cravings and hunger pangs? Sure you would. So, tell your subconscious mind that.

What else would you like? How about finding it easy to follow your preferred dietary program?

Or ... how about feeling totally filled up and satisfied every time after eating a right amount of food, or the amount prescribed by your preferred dietary program?

Or ... how about finding right foods, or the foods prescribed by your dietary program, to be tasty and satisfying?

Or ... how about finding wrong foods, or the foods prohibited by your dietary program, to be unappealing and tasteless?

Or ... how about each meal turning out to be a "healthy-meal victory" and you having a great feeling of satisfaction after each one?

Or ... how about finding your daily exercise activity to be enjoyable and invigorating?

Or ... how about your subconscious mind reminding you to do all five daily actions of the Weight Success Method, plus automatically performing every action described in the Weight Success Benefits Directive?

Would you like one or more of these things to happen? Sure you would. So, tell your subconscious mind exactly what you want it to help make happen in the upcoming day. Doing this takes less than 60 seconds. But the results can astound.

Try Resting-mind Mode

Now here's an optional tip for possibly enhancing the impact of your upcoming-day descriptions. Your conscious mind mainly functions in two modes: awake and sleeping. In the awake mode it's active. As such, it's busy receiving and processing stimuli and responding to events going on around you. During this time it directs most or all of your words and actions. We call this *awake-mind mode.*

In the sleeping mode your conscious mind is inactive. As such, it pays little or no attention to stimuli around you, except that which it interprets as being an emergency.

However, you have periods where you aren't completely sleeping but also not fully functioning in awake-mind mode. These periods often occur when you're in the process of either waking up or falling asleep, or between awake-mind and sleeping modes. For reference purpose we'll call such periods *resting-mind mode.*

Resting-mind mode usually lasts for a short period, like a few minutes. But sometimes it can go longer. It mainly occurs when you're (a) drifting off to sleep, (b) waking up in the night, such as before going to the bathroom or otherwise arising for something, (c) going back to sleep in the night (such as after going to the bathroom), and (d) waking up in the morning, or when you're awake but haven't yet opened your eyes and arisen from bed.

During resting-mind mode your conscious mind is functioning but it's not focusing on and dealing with stimuli and events of the world around you. So, what's the difference between awake-mind mode and resting-mind mode? In awake-mind mode your conscious mind is mainly focusing on the events of the outer world. In resting-mind mode it's mainly focusing on the events of the inner world, or the activity of your subconscious mind.

A unique feature of resting-mind mode is the opportunity for enhanced communication between you and your subconscious mind. For some reason, messages sent to your subconscious mind during resting-mind mode often have a stronger impact on your subconscious mind. It's as if your subconscious mind focuses on these messages more intently, or views them as being of higher importance.

If you find communicating to your subconscious mind during resting-mind mode to be effective *and* you'd like to do this type of communication at times other than at night or in the morning, or during sleep time, you can easily do so. Just do this. Close your eyes, relax your conscious mind, and begin silently talking to your subconscious mind. The more relaxed you are and the more your conscious mind is detached from focusing on external stimuli, the easier and more effective the communication will be. Becoming proficient at this is easy to do. All you do is practice it a few times, and deliver positive reinforcement to yourself after your conscious

mind follows instructions and goes into resting-mind mode.

How to Get Input from Your Subconscious

Here's an additional thing you can do in resting-mind mode. It's not directly related to weight control, but it's something you might be able to apply for personal benefit. (Note: I've been using it for years in creative pursuits, such as, for example, in creating inventions and patents and also in book writing.) Basically, it's an easy way to get timely input — mainly, ideas and suggestions — from your subconscious mind. Messages from your subconscious mind seem to come through more distinctly in resting-mind mode than in awake-mind mode. Here's how to do it.

First, put your conscious mind into resting-mind mode. Then, to get an answer or idea on a specific topic, pose a simple clearly-worded question to your subconscious mind. Make the question as clear and specific as possible. Why? Because your subconscious typically can't or won't respond to a vague ambiguous question.

Often your subconscious will send back an answer almost instantly. If it doesn't, set a deadline for it to deliver a response — like, for example, "by 9:00 a.m. tomorrow morning."

The message that comes back from your subconscious mind will likely be in the form of a fleeting thought, or idea or realization, or phrase, or image, or feeling, or hunch, or musical lyric, or memory of a past event. At this point it's up to you to interpret what it means. Much of the time the meaning is crystal clear; it's a "do this" type of message. Other times it's symbolic, so it requires some interpretation. And, now and then it seems inexplicable. When this happens ask your subconscious mind to send a clarifying message, which it usually will do. Or, rephrase the question. Oftentimes when you get an incomprehensible response it's because you posed a confusing question. To get a simple, specific, unambiguous answer, pose a simple, specific, unambiguous question. Lastly, *thank* your subconscious mind for sending the answer.

To get maximum benefit from this process, keep a pad and pencil by your bedside or chairside, and also a small table light or flashlight for night use. When your subconscious mind sends some insightful or useful info, open your eyes, turn on the light, and write down the message on the pad. When finished writing, lay down, close your eyes, and go back to resting-mind mode. If you like, you can continue the communication where you left off.

I've found that the best pencil for this is an automatic pencil with erasure. The best pad is a 6-by-9 inch steno pad with a wire coil at the top. You can handily store the automatic pencil by sliding it into the end of the wire coil, with the pencil's clip engaging the wire. If you use this process often you might find it helpful to put the date at the top of the first page of each session. This makes it easier to refer back to a message at a later date.

> ## MOTIVATOR 4:
> ### Day-end Thanks
> **At the end of the day, right before going to sleep, thank your subconscious mind for at least one desired action it performed that day.**

A "desired action" would be any action that assisted you with achieving right eating or healthy-weight living. Another name for this is "weight success action."

Thanking your subconscious mind after it performs a desired action, along with telling it to repeat that action in the future, motivates it to repeat the action in the future. This dynamic is a key factor in daily Actions 2A and 5.

Unfortunately, most people are oblivious to the desired actions their subconscious mind performs throughout each day. As such, they never thank it for these actions. The result: They miss out on a big opportunity to motivate their subconscious mind to *more frequently* perform desired actions. But, you can go a long way toward rectifying this situation by

applying this Motivator 4. Here's how. After going to bed for the night, close your eyes and relax your mind. Then do these two things.

FIRST, mentally review the past day. In doing this, identify one or more specific weight success actions performed by your subconscious mind. Note: When your subconscious mind does any of the actions described in your Weight Success Benefits Directive, that's a *weight success action*.

SECOND, deliver thanks to your subconscious mind for having performed this desired action. For this, deliver a short Thank You, Keep It Up message. You can deliver your thanks either by speaking silently in your mind or by speaking aloud. Note: whispering counts as speaking aloud. Do it whatever way feels most natural and meaningful at the time. Doing this Motivator 4 takes less than 30 seconds. But the results can be powerful.

> ## MOTIVATOR 5:
> ### Benefits Visualization
> **For at least 60 seconds, visualize one of your exciting weight success benefits as an accomplished fact, at least once a day.**

In delivering your Weight Success Benefits Directive (for Daily Action 3, page 50) you briefly visualize the attainment of a weight success benefit. With this Motivator 5 you do it more in-depth. Here's how. Sit in a relaxing chair or lay in bed, close your eyes, and visualize one of your exciting weight success benefits as an accomplished fact. That is, visualize the benefit being fully achieved and you enjoying it that very moment. Mentally fill the scene with pleasant details. Create a good feeling in yourself — this is important. Visualize for at least a minute.

Also, do at least one visualization a day. You can visualize the same weight success benefit each time *or* you can visualize a different benefit each time — your choice.

Visualization exists in two forms: still image and moving image. A still-image visualization is a mental picture of a single situation or thing, like a mental photograph. A moving-image visualization is a mental picture of a moving action or event, like a mental video or movie. This mental movie can be in either third person or first person. In **third** person you're *viewing* yourself performing the action, like watching a movie. In **first** person you're imagining yourself being in the process of *doing* the action, like making the movie. Some persons believe the first-person approach is more effective than the third-person. Do it whichever way creates the most enjoyable feeling.

MOTIVATOR 6:
Goal Reminders

View goal-reminding images each day.

Each day view images and messages pertaining to your healthy-weight goal and ongoing realization of that goal. Whenever you see such an image it causes three events to occur.

First, it momentarily focuses your mind, including subconscious mind, on the continuing realization of that goal.

Second, it reminds you to do all five Daily Actions of the Weight Success Method that day.

Third, it reminds you of your substantial accomplishment in sustaining ongoing daily realization of your healthy-weight goal. This can — and should — give you a surging feeling of joy and pride.

These three events motivate you and your subconscious mind to make that day be a Weight Success Day — that is, a day that contributes to creating weight success.

So, what might you use for visual reminders of your healthy-weight goal and of your ongoing realization of that goal? For illustration, here are three examples of visual goal reminders:

1 – A prominently displayed note or sign depicting the number of years (months or weeks) you've been living in your healthy-weight range. On page 13 is an example of such a note, which is pinned to my bulletin board and is viewed by me every day. It's a *very* powerful reminder.

2 – A prominently displayed Win-Day Calendar, which is described in the *Handy Extra Tools* chapter (p. 174).

3 – A prominently displayed Weight Success Actions Scorecard, which is described in the *Handy Extra Tools* chapter (p. 174).

Those are three examples. It's likely you can create visual goal and progress reminders of your own design. Finally, "post" your visual reminders not only on paper but also on your digital devices. In short, put them "all over," so that you see them *throughout each day.*

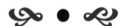

Most people underestimate the faculties of their subconscious mind. And, their subconscious mind — always eager to fulfill expectations — responds in accordance with the underestimation.

CHAPTER 14: How to Adapt the Weight Success Method to Fix Problems

Be dogged in fixing weight management problems, and you'll *succeed* at surmounting every one.

THE SECOND PART of the Weight Success Method (p. **44**) provides exact procedures for the five daily actions. But in spots it tells you to feel free to improvise. This is for two reasons: (1) so you might make the Method more closely fit your situation, and (2) so that if you confront a special problem — such as a troublesome eating urge, craving, or habit — you might create a special solution that enables you to more readily surmount that problem.

To help you apply reason #2, this chapter gives eleven special problem resolution tactics, any of which you might apply for helping resolve an occasional special problem that could arise.

TACTIC 1: In Daily Action 2A–Reinforcement (p. **45**), when delivering the Thank You, Keep It Up message, include a special instruction to your subconscious mind that tells it what you want done regarding resolution of the special problem.

TACTIC 2: In Daily Action 3–Benefits Directive (p. **50**), when delivering the Weight Success Benefits Directive include some ad lib instruction to your subconscious mind that tells it what you want done regarding resolution of the special problem.

TACTIC 3: For the Weight Success Benefits Directive (p. **52**), write up an additional healthy-weight action. Word it so it tells your subconscious mind what to do regarding resolving the special problem on an ongoing basis. Make it action #6 and incorporate it into the Directive after action #5. You can write it in or type it up and tape it in.

TACTIC 4: In Daily Action 5–Guided Eating (p. **56**), apply a custom guided-eating self-talk statement. In Step 1 of the Action (the Communication step), two sample statements are provided. But for resolving a special eating-related problem you could create your own customized self-talk statement for neutralizing that problem.

Upcoming Tactics #5–9 are adaptations of the six optional mind motivators described in the *Six More Mind Motivators* chapter (p. **110**).

TACTIC 5: Apply Motivator 1: High-frequency Goal Statement (p. **110**). For this, say your Healthy-weight Goal Statement a hundred times a day. Sometimes an intense focus on the ultimate goal of your weight success journey can have the effect of neutralizing, or "drowning," a special problem.

TACTIC 6: Apply Motivator 2: Backup Depiction Statements (p. **110**). For this, create a custom backup depiction statement aimed at neutralizing the special problem. Make it describe an action or outcome you want your subconscious to do, or describe some affirmation you want your whole mind to take heed of and actualize. Say the statement many times per day.

TACTIC 7: Apply Motivator 3: Upcoming-day Description (p. **112**). For this, do an upcoming-day depiction that describes the special problem being resolved, and what it will be like after it's resolved.

TACTIC 8: Apply Motivator 4: Day-end Thanks (p. **114**). For this, at the end of the day reflect back on the special problem. Did you, or your subconscious mind, perform any action that amounted to progress in resolving the problem? If so, deliver appreciation and thanks to your subconscious mind (use a type of Thank You, Keep It Up message).

TACTIC 9: Apply Motivator 5: Benefits Visualization (p. **114**). For this, use the visualization technique described for Motivator 5 and visualize the problem resolved and you enjoying it.

TACTIC 10: Ask your subconscious mind to tell you the best way to solve the problem. To do this, use the technique described in the section titled "How to Get Input from Your Subconscious" (p. **113**).

TACTIC 11: Ask God to disclose to you an insight, tactic, or opportunity you might use for resolving the special problem and, thereby, creating easier lifelong healthy-weight living. This method consists of three parts: Communicate, Believe, Appreciate. (Sound familiar?) It can be done anytime, but a particularly good time is before going to sleep for the night.

Three Steps to Getting and Using Input from God

Here's what to do.

Step 1 – COMMUNICATE. *Communicate to God the full situation regarding the problem you want to resolve, and then request God to disclose a solution to you.* ✍ As you convey the message, imagine, or assume, that God, or God's spirit, is invisibly present in the room with you at that very moment. Then, include the following information in your communication:

(1) an *exact description* of the problem you want to resolve,

(2) an expression of *strong desire* for God to disclose to you an insight, tactic, or opportunity that, if employed by you, would resolve the problem,

(3) the *reason why* you want the problem resolved, or how having the problem resolved will greatly benefit you and your life,

(4) an expression of your firm *belief* that God will be acting on your request,

and then after doing parts 1–4,

(5) *ask God* to please disclose the input you're seeking by a certain time (like, for example, "by 9 a.m. tomorrow morning").

Step 2 – BELIEVE. *Fully believe that God will be following through on your request and that the input will be forthcoming within the requested time.* ✍ Hold this belief both while making the request

and afterward as well. Also, keep these three points in mind:

(1) God's response or input can come at any time, including (a) immediately, like within a minute after making the request, or (b) just before the specified deadline, or (c) in a dream, or (d) while you're waking up or right after waking up.

(2) When the response comes, immediately write it down on a piece of paper (or perhaps on a digital device), so keep paper and pencil or digital device handy — that is, by your bedside (if you don't write it down you'll likely find it hard to remember later, or the next morning).

(3) The message that comes back from God can be in the form of a fleeting thought, or idea or realization, or phrase, or image, or feeling, or hunch, or musical lyric, or memory of a past event. At this point it's up to you to interpret what it means. Much of the time the meaning is crystal clear; it's a "do this" type of message. Other times it's symbolic, so it requires some interpretation. And, now and then it seems inexplicable. When this happens ask God to send a clarifying message.

Step 3 – APPRECIATE. *When the requested input comes, thank God for it; then <u>proceed to apply it</u>.* ✍ If this insight involves ongoing action of some sort, incorporate the action into your daily application of the Weight Success Method.

> NOTE: To the best of my conjecture, God doesn't get involved in directing a person to impose harm or negative consequences on their self or on another person. So, when I say "apply God's input" I'm not suggesting you pursue something that's rude or illegal or immoral or potentially harmful to you or to someone else, or that would constitute an imposition or trespass on someone or their property. If such a thought should come to mind, convert it into a version that's courteous, legal, moral, and non-harmful to you and others; then pursue this legal, harmless version. In other words, pursue only harm-free activities.

As you now know, the key to succeeding at lifelong healthy-weight living is:

Do Weight Success Actions <u>every day</u>.

For maximal effectiveness in doing this, be creative in applying the Weight Success Method for surmounting any problem that arises, and don't hesitate to use every available resource and Tactic (#1–11 on prior pages) for realizing your healthy-weight goal.

<u>This</u> is how weight success is most easily and enjoyably accomplished.

CHAPTER 15: Achieving Exercise Success

An exercise program could expedite healthy-weight living, but it's not a requirement. By applying the Weight Success Method you can live at your desired weight without exercising, although you might need to eat a little less food to do it.

MOST PERSONS view exercise as a "non-essential" to achieving good health and a good life. So they don't do it on a regular basis. Truth is, for most of us exercise enhances virtually every aspect of our being, for the entire duration of our life. Few activities benefit us as much as daily exercise does. Plus it does one other interesting thing: It can make weight reduction and weight management *easier*.

Also, before beginning a new exercise program or making a major change to a present program you should consult with your physician to ensure you're physically capable of performing the program without personal harm or medical issues.

Seven Keys to Exercise Success

Use these seven keys for starting, sticking with, and enjoying the daily exercise activity of your choice. These pointers apply to virtually every type of exercise.

KEY 1: *Pursue exercise activities you enjoy doing.* ❧ When you don't enjoy doing a particular exercise you likely won't stick with it. When you *do* enjoy doing a particular exercise you have a greater chance of succeeding with it. Also, you don't need to limit yourself to doing the same type of exercise every day. To avoid boredom, have a "stable" of exercises you can choose from. My exercise stable, for example, includes walking, weight-resistance workout, bicycling, and a recumbent training bike.

KEY 2: *Start small and build up gradually.* ❧ The biggest mistake most people make when undertaking an exercise program is they start wrong. They (a) attempt too much in the first day or week or (b) build up too quickly or (c) do both. In doing this they either sustain an injury or become so exhausted they mentally burn out. So start small, build up gradually. That's how you succeed at exercise.

KEY 3: *Use the right technique and gear.* ❧ For virtually every type of exercise there's a right way and a wrong way to do it. The wrong way almost always creates problems, sometimes big ones. So, learn the correct way to perform your chosen exercise. You might get a book or DVD on it. Also, using the right gear and apparel can help. In short, don't take chances with wrong technique or gear. Avoid problems by doing it the right way from the start.

KEY 4: *Record your exercise sessions.* ❧ On a calendar or a chart, record what you did and when you did it. This gives you added opportunity to feel good about what you're doing. It's called positive reinforcement. It motivates you to continue doing the thing that made you feel good.

KEY 5: *Keep it fun.* ❧ If a particular exercise session is turning out to be not-fun you might end it early. Don't force yourself to have a bad experience. This only de-motivates you in the future. Also, if your chosen exercise activity begins to grow stale or become not-fun, modify it to be fun again. Or, adopt a different type of exercise. Do whatever it takes to keep your exercising fun ... or, at least, to keep it from becoming an unpleasant experience.

KEY 6: *Make doing your chosen exercise a top priority.* ❧ When doing your exercise isn't a top priority it always ends up being bumped out of line by some other "more important thing." So, you end up not sticking with it — or, at best, doing it hit-and-miss. To succeed at exercising you must view getting your regular exercise as being mandatory, not optional. Scheduling it for a certain timeslot in the day can help. For many persons, doing it at the start of the day works best.

KEY 7: *Try to do at least some exercise every day, or most days, of the week.* ❧ To succeed at exercise, exercise must be a habit with you. To maintain exercise as a habit it helps to engage in some form of exercise at least several days a week.

How to Make Yourself Start and Stay with It

Every activity has both an upside and a downside. The upside is that aspect of the activity that you like or enjoy. The downside is that aspect that you dislike or don't enjoy. When the downside looms large in your mind you find it hard to make yourself do the activity.

Often, the hardest part to doing an exercise program is making yourself take the first step. This results from the perceived downside — or hassle, aggravation, annoyance, discomfort — attached to doing the exercise. Which means, if the downside were to be reduced to insignificance, *you would start doing the exercise!* So, the key to beginning an exercise program is reduce the downside to insignificance.

You can use an easy 2-step technique for reducing the downside to insignificance — and, thereby, making yourself start and stick with a particular exercise:

1. Reduce the exercise to a miniscule amount, and start at that amount;

2. Increase the exercise amount in miniscule increments and very gradually over time.

How to Enhance the Upside

The above technique reduces the downside of exercising. Now what you also should do is enhance the upside. You can do this one or both of two ways.

One, before each exercise session deliver a short directive to your mind. In this directive tell your mind to make the exercise feel enjoyable. That is, tell it to minimize any emotional discomfort you might feel from exercising. Also, tell it to cause you

to derive a feeling of pleasure and satisfaction from the act of exercising — both while exercising and afterward. To help make this happen, while exercising visualize yourself being in possession of one or more of your weight success benefits, which are the items listed in the benefits section of your Weight Success Benefits Directive.

Two, after the exercising deliver to your self — or your mind — a Thank You, Keep It Up message. Thank it for reminding you to do the exercise. Also thank it for assisting you with making the exercise enjoyable. In short, after each exercise session deliver to yourself a generous dose of positive self-reinforcement. The main idea is to generate a good feeling after each session.

Concluding Summary

Regular exercise is one of the most beneficial activities you can engage in. One of those benefits is easier weight loss and weight control. You can enhance your chance of exercise success by doing certain things. It works like this.

Seven Keys to Exercise Success

1. Pursue exercise activities you enjoy doing.
2. Start small and build up gradually.
3. Use the right technique and gear.
4. Record your exercise sessions.
5. Keep it fun, or at least keep it from being unpleasant.
6. Make doing your chosen exercise a top priority.
7. Try to do at least some exercise every day (or most days).

Results in exercise success which, in turn, creates numerous benefits including easier weight loss and weight control.

Two Types of Weight-control Exercise: (1) Pushing through a daily workout, (2) pushing away from the table. Type 1 works for some people; type 2 works for all. But do both, if you like.

CHAPTER 16: Escaping Schadenfreude

(and also escaping reverse-schadenfreude)

SCHADENFREUDE is a German word. Literally, it means "damage-joy" (schaden = damage; freude = joy). But a dictionary-type definition would be: *delight, joy, or pleasure derived from seeing or hearing about someone else's troubles, failures, or misfortunes.*

So, what does this have to do with healthy-weight living? More than you might imagine. You might assume that your family and friends would want to see you succeed in your weight success journey. You might assume that once you've made the decision to change your life from overweight living to healthy-weight living that they'd be cheering you on. You might assume that after you've switched from wrong eating to right eating they'd take joy in you doing this, and delight in hearing about your progress, and want to encourage and assist you. You might assume that as your body slowly morphs from overweight to right weight that they'd be happy to see you that way, and offer sincere compliments and encouraging words.

Some family members and friends will respond that way. But also it's likely some will not. Their typical response will be no response. What's more, the more progress you make the more "no response" there will be.

Now, you might assume that the reason for this "no response" is that these people have no interest in what you're doing, no interest in learning about what's happening in your life.

But probably that's not the case. They likely have considerable interest in hearing about what's happening with you. But it's not an interest in hearing about what you're succeeding with; it's an interest in hearing about what you're struggling and failing with. Which means, as regards your weight success journey, these people will show little interest in hearing about your progress and successes but will have keen interest in learning of your troubles and setbacks and, perhaps most of all, your ultimate failure.

Why do some people respond this way? Schadenfreude! Every time they hear about how you might be struggling with losing weight or with maintaining your desired weight it creates a pleasurable feeling in them. Further, every time they hear about how you might be succeeding in your weight-loss program it creates a not-so-pleasurable feeling in them. I call this *reverse-schadenfreude.* (I don't know what the German word for "success-misery" would be.) In short, for some people your weight management failure = their joy; your weight management success = their misery. So they love hearing about your weight struggles and setbacks, and hate hearing about your weight progress and accomplishments.

What's the most productive way to deal with this perverse situation? Do these four things.

1 — As regards the "no-positive-response folks," realize that schadenfreude and reverse-schadenfreude are what is driving their response. Meaning, recognize that their negative response to your weight management pursuit is not because of you but because of some deviant schadenfreude (or reverse-schadenfreude) dynamic they carry in their head.

2 — Ignore the no-response/negative response of the "schadenfreuders." Meaning, don't let this response deter or discourage you. Realize that this is just the way some people are. Bear in mind that (a) you're on the right track with your pursuit of healthy-weight living and (b) they're on some other track with their seeming inability to view the pursuit of healthy-weight living in a positive light.

3 — Embrace those family members and friends who view your weight success journey in a positive light. Maintain, or perhaps build, your relationship with them.

4 — If you feel overwhelmed or discouraged by some peoples' negative response to your weight success journey, consider joining a dietary program that involves interaction with others — that is, with instructors and co-dieters who provide encouragement and support. This will offset the potentially-discouraging negative response of those who secretly desire to see you struggle with creating healthy-weight living.

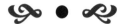

Always, always bear in mind:
Despite what anyone might say or believe, you <u>have</u> the capability to live your life in your healthy-weight range *and* you have the capability to do it <u>easily</u>, or at least way more easily than you, or they, might be imagining.

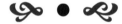

Just Keep Doing Essential

Weight Success Actions

Every Day ... and Lifelong
Weight Success will be Yours.

CHAPTER 17: Why the Weight Success Method is Enjoyable

Most people assume weight management is painful. But, actually, doing the Weight Success Method is *enjoyable* and *uplifting*.

SHORTLY after starting the Weight Success Method in 2007 I made an eye-opening discovery. I realized that the *process* of doing the Method can be enjoyable and gratifying in itself. Here's how it happens.

Enjoyment from the PROCESS

All five daily actions of the Weight Success Method produce enjoyment.

Daily Action 1 – Weighing (p. 44)

You might find this hard to believe, but it's true. Each day I look forward to my daily weighing. Now, some people might deride this. They could say "you're weight obsessed" or "you're vain and self-absorbed over how you look."

But such conclusions miss the point. I don't spend time obsessing over body weight. And, I'm not one to be vain and self-absorbed over personal appearance, or at least no more than anyone else.

Rather, what I *am* absorbed with is giving myself opportunity to become the finest person I can be and to create the most beneficial life I can create. This includes realizing the many benefits that come with living in my healthy-weight range. In short, becoming the finest person I can be and creating the most beneficial life I can create is a top priority of mine.

So, it's obvious why I enjoy weighing myself each day. It's because my daily weighing gives me timely feedback on the daily progress I'm making toward realization of one of my top priorities. I find this to be enjoyable. Indeed, not only do I find it enjoyable I find it motivating and uplifting, as well — a great way to start a day.

Now, you might be thinking: What about when you get a scale reading that shows your weight being above your healthy-weight range? How do you feel then?

Well, naturally, I feel disappointment. But in no way am I sad or discouraged. I view it as an opportunity — an opportunity to gain extra enjoyment at the next day's weighing. Whenever I get a desired weight reading the day after getting an undesired one, or return to my healthy-weight range after straying from it, it doesn't just make me feel good, it makes me feel *very* good. So, on the infrequent occasion when my weight slips outside my healthy-weight range I take immediate, vigorous corrective action in the next 24 or 48 hours (Daily Action 2B). This immediately brings my body weight back into line, which brings me extra enjoyment at a subsequent day's weighing.

To add to this discussion I note that most persons hate stepping onto a scale. That's because it too often results in a painful experience. But this painful experience occurs because they're doing weighing and weight control the wrong way.

By applying the approach described in Daily Action 1, I actually derive enjoyment from daily weighing. And, in turn, this enjoyment makes it easier for me to motivate my mind to stick with my healthy-weight living activities and program. In short, doing Daily Action 1 is an enjoyable, motivating, uplifting experience for me. It can be this way for you, too.

Daily Action 2A – Reinforcement (p. 45)

Each time I deliver the Thank You, Keep It Up message after the daily weighing, I deliver it with happiness and exuberance. I make it a joyous moment. This, in turn, builds on the great feeling I derived from getting the positive feedback, or desired weight reading, that came with the daily weighing. In short, doing Daily Action 2A is an enjoyable, motivating, uplifting experience.

Daily Action 2B – Correction (p. 48)

Perhaps it's hard to see how doing Daily Action 2B could be enjoyable. But, believe it or not, I actually derive pleasure and gratification from it. It's all in the perspective.

If I view doing this action as "proof that I'm a weight-control failure" then, as you might expect, I feel badly. But, on the other hand, when I view it as "proof that I'm a weight-control winner" I feel good. A winner, after all, isn't someone who never experiences setbacks or makes mistakes or misses the mark now and then. Rather, a winner is one who learns from mistakes, bounces back after setbacks, and persists in spite of missteps. More precisely, a winner is one who, after a setback, ratchets up their focus and intensity to the point where they surmount the setback and, once having done so, emerges as a stronger, smarter person than they were before the setback. That's the viewpoint and approach I take when doing Daily Action 2B. It works every time — meaning, every time it puts me instantly back on track *and* generates a good feeling, too.

So, I pursue Daily Action 2B with intensity and resoluteness. I view it as a positive experience. And, I view it as proof that I'm a winner in general and a healthy-weight winner in particular. Approaching it this way makes doing Daily Action 2B enjoyable and motivating.

What this comes down to is positive approach to a setback versus negative approach. With a positive approach — described above — the correction process is pleasurable and successful. With a negative approach — opposite of the above — the correction process usually turns out to be painful and often unsuccessful. Plus, applying the positive approach requires no more time and effort than applying a negative one. So, I opt for the positive perspective — and derive enjoyment and benefit from it.

Daily Action 3 – Benefits Directive (p. 50)

In terms of time, Daily Action 3 requires the most commitment. It involves setting aside two to three minutes a day of dedicated time for delivering the Weight Success Benefits Directive. So one could view it as being a time-consuming inconvenience. And when something's viewed as an inconvenience it tends to be non-enjoyable.

But it needn't be this way. I've found that delivering the Directive can be an enjoyable experience if I do one or more of these three things.

First, I act as-if my mind — in particular my subconscious mind — is right then, as I'm reading the Directive, in the process of acting on every instruction I'm giving it. Which means the present day is going to be a right-eating day — also known as healthy-eating day. This is a pleasure-producing thought.

Second, I bear in mind the many weight success benefits I gain from living in my healthy-weight range. This is another pleasure-producing thought. These benefits are cited in the Directive.

Third, I apply a creative delivery technique now and then, as described in action #7 of the Seven Actions for Delivering the Directive for Maximum Effect (p. **87**). Indeed, the cliché is correct: Variety is the spice of life.

Doing any of these three things increases the enjoyment I derive from Daily Action 3. It makes the action less like a chore and more like a pleasure.

Daily Action 4 – Goal Statement (p. 54)

Saying the Healthy-weight Goal Statement 25 — or 40 or 50 or 100 — times a day might seem like repetitive drudgery. And drudgery isn't fun. But it doesn't have to be this way. There are three things I do to change this potential drudgery into enjoyment.

First, each time I say my Healthy-weight Goal Statement I *act as-if* I am at that very moment the person depicted in the statement. That is, I act as-if I'm "the person of my healthy weight" and one who's "healthy, happy, and doing great." Or, put another way, whenever I say my Healthy-weight Goal Statement I realize that I am, indeed, the actual person depicted in the Statement. This imparts a good feeling within me.

Second, as I'm saying the Statement I call to mind one or two exciting weight success benefits.

And then I act as-if my mind is right then in the process of actualizing these benefits with every iteration of my Healthy-weight Goal Statement. This also gives me a good feeling.

Third, I change up my delivery style from time to time. For example, the Statement can be said rapidly or slowly. And different words can be emphasized at different times.

Doing these three things, especially the first two, make Daily Action 4 enjoyable, motivating, and uplifting.

Daily Action 5 – Guided Eating (p. 56)

Daily Action 5 involves applying the Guided Eating Process to each eating session. The Guided Eating Process consists of Communicate, Believe, Appreciate. In acronym form, I call it the C-B-A process (which is A-B-C in reverse). To review, doing this process involves these three steps.

Communicate Step. As the eating begins — and perhaps during the meal too — I deliver guided-eating self-talk to my self, or my mind.

Believe Step. As I'm eating I hold the belief, and also act as-if, my mind is right then, at that very moment, in the process of performing the actions described in my guided-eating self-talk; so I'm on the lookout for a stop-eating signal, which usually includes the full-stomach feeling.

Appreciate Step. If a stop-eating signal comes I thank my mind — or, more specifically, my subconscious mind — for sending the signal; then I follow the signal — that is, I stop eating. When I do this the urge to continue eating immediately begins to fade away.

Now we come to the main point. Doing this 3-step process — especially the third step — gives me a feeling of accomplishment. It makes me realize that I control my eating and my eating isn't controlling me. And, this makes me feel good. It makes me feel like a healthy-weight winner. I like that feeling. It's enjoyable, gratifying, and uplifting.

Summary of Process Enjoyment

So to sum up, here are the six kinds of enjoyment I derive from the process of doing the Weight Success Method.

1 – *Enjoyment from Daily Progress.* Each time I get a desired weight reading when doing my daily weighing (Daily Action 1) it tells me I've achieved yet another day of progress toward the further realization of lifelong healthy-weight living. I find this to be enjoyable, motivating, and uplifting.

2 – *Enjoyment from Daily Reinforcement.* Each time that I deliver and receive positive self-reinforcement I find it to be enjoyable, motivating, and uplifting. This comes from delivering an exuberant Thank You, Keep It Up message to my self — or my mind — after each desired weight reading (Daily Action 2A).

3 – *Enjoyment from Triumphing over Adversity or Setback.* Each time that I do Daily Action 2B I triumph over a setback and also derive a benefit from the process. Doing this I find to be enjoyable, motivating, and uplifting.

4 – *Enjoyment from Being Director of My Eating.* In any given eating situation, either I'm the director of my eating *or* my eating is the director of me. I accomplish being director of my eating by applying the Weight Success Method, and especially by doing Daily Actions 3 and 5. I find that being director of my eating is enjoyable, motivating, and uplifting.

5 – *Enjoyment from Focusing on an Exciting Ultimate Goal.* My days seem to go better and obstacles and annoyances seem to be smaller when I'm focusing on an exciting ultimate goal. Doing the five daily actions of the Weight Success Method focuses me each day on one of my ultimate goals — specifically, being the person of my healthy weight and living my life in my healthy-weight range. Doing Daily Action 4 keeps me focused on this goal. I find this to be enjoyable, motivating, and uplifting.

6 – *Enjoyment from Viewing Myself as a Winner.* I like viewing myself as a winner. Or, more directly, I like being a winner. And what's a winner? A winner is someone who performs winning actions. The Weight Success Method is full of opportunities for winning actions. Each time I do one of the five daily actions I'm performing a winning action. Also, each time I do one of the actions described in any of the optional chapters in Section B (especially Chapter 27) I'm doing a winning action. I find doing winning actions and feeling like a winner to be enjoyable, motivating, and uplifting.

To sum up, doing the five daily actions of the Weight Success Method involves interacting with my self in a way that motivates my mind — including subconscious mind — to steer me toward living in my healthy-weight range. For the reasons just described, I find this interaction process enjoyable, motivating, and uplifting.

Enjoyment from the OUTCOME

Along with deriving enjoyment from the process of doing the five daily actions, I also get it from the outcome. This outcome manifests in two forms: general and specific.

The general outcome is: living my life in my healthy-weight range. Presently, the act of putting one's weight into a healthy-weight range and then *maintaining* it there for the rest of one's life is a rare accomplishment. Which means any person who's accomplishing it is a healthy-weight high-achiever. Living my life as such a person I find to be enjoyable, motivating, and uplifting.

From this general outcome arises a specific outcome: the realization of my weight success benefits. The benefit I find to be most motivating and uplifting is benefit #1: a greater chance of living healthier longer, or greater chance of living free of debilitating accidents, illnesses, diseases, and bodily malfunction.

Now here's a big point. Enjoyment from benefits comes two ways: (1) from *actualization* of the benefit and (2) from being *aware* of the benefit on a daily basis. Doing the Weight Success Method, especially Daily Actions 3 and 4, maintains my awareness of my weight success benefits on a daily

basis. As a result, I derive substantial enjoyment and motivation from my weight success benefits.

To sum up, I enjoy the outcome of the Weight Success Method *and* I enjoy the process of creating the outcome. So, in terms of enjoyment, gratification, and fulfillment, the Weight Success Method is a double-win. This double-win — plus the fact that creating it typically requires less than eight minutes of dedicated time per day — is why I continue doing the Method day after day, year after year. It's also why I decided to publish it in this book.

Bad Pleasure | Good Pleasure

For the first six decades of my life I held a certain limiting assumption. The assumption was that the main purpose of my life was to do things that resulted in personal enjoyment, happiness, success, and fulfillment. This assumption seemed inherently obvious to me.

But there was a slippery little question lurking in the bushes of my mind. That being: What, exactly, are the activities that (will) result in creating personal enjoyment, happiness, success, and fulfillment? In a sense, I spent the first 60 years of my life trying to find the answer to that question. And the answer eluded me.

Then, one day while writing the original weight management book — which, believe it or not, spanned a period of over six years (yes, there were numerous versions and re-writes) — the answer came.

And, what came is this. The purpose of my life is to (a) strive to become the finest person I'm capable of being, (b) strive to create the most beneficial life I'm capable of creating, and (c) help as many others as I can to do the same. I then realized that performing these three actions is the reason my life exists — and perhaps the reason why all human lives exist. Then I further realized that it's through performance of these three actions that I — and perhaps humankind — experience maximal peace, love, joy, and fulfillment in life.

After that, I realized that all pleasures and pursuits can be divided into two groups: (1) those that assist me in performing those three actions and (2) those that hinder me in performing those actions.

For identification purposes I dubbed the first group *good pleasures and pursuits* and the second group *bad pleasures and pursuits*. Alternatively, these two groups could be called *productive* pleasures and pursuits and *counterproductive* pleasures and pursuits.

And then I realized that a pivotal factor in determining the course of my life were the decisions I had made regarding what pleasures to pursue. And, further, I realized it was not only a deciding factor in *my* life but was also a factor in determining the prior history, and perhaps the "future history," of humankind.

All this raised a question. When we humans confront an either/or decision regarding pursuing an activity that yields a bad pleasure versus an activity that yields a good pleasure, why do we sometimes, or perhaps much of the time, opt to pursue the bad activity? It's because of this. The pleasures derived from performing an activity in the bad activity group tend to be large at the start; while the pleasures derived from performing an activity in the good activity group tend to be smaller at the start. So, we're often motivated to pursue a bad activity over an opposing good activity because the bad activity affords the most pleasure *right now*.

There is, however, an additional distinction between these two types of pleasure-producing activities. Although the bad activity often yields the largest immediate pleasure this pleasure tends to diminish over time — and often eventually diminishes to the point of being a "negative pleasure," or pain and handicap.

On the other hand, although the good activity might yield a smaller immediate pleasure this pleasure tends to expand over time — and often continues expanding to the end of a person's life — and ultimately provides large lasting benefits.

So, why have I included this discussion in a book on eating and weight management? It's because, like so many aspects of human life, eating and weight management come down to "choosing our pleasures," or deciding whether to (a) pursue a counterproductive activity that produces a large immediate pleasure but eventually creates a large future penalty or (b) pursue a productive activity that produces a smaller immediate pleasure but eventually yields large future benefits.

As pertains to this book, what I'm talking about is the choice between overeating and non-overeating. Overeating affords, or appears to afford, the opportunity for greater eating pleasure in the present but brings on long-term penalty and suffering that *hinders* me in my pursuit to become the finest person I can be and create the most beneficial life I can create.

Non-overeating, on the other hand, might afford lesser eating pleasure in the present but it brings major long-term benefits, those benefits being my weight success benefits. In doing so, non-overeating *assists* me in becoming the finest person I can be and in creating the most beneficial life I can create.

Plus, it enables me to "help others do the same." And how does it enable me to help others? Many people hold the belief that how they live their life affects only them. But that's self-deceiving rationalization, and grossly incorrect. *Their life impacts every life around them,* whether they want it to or not. What they do that's not-so-good inflicts not-so-good impact on those around them. And what they do that's good bestows good on those around them. This is especially the case when one is a parent, grandparent, spouse, sibling, or close friend.

One of the most powerful ways we impact the lives of those around us, for better or for worse, is by *how* we live our life. Like it or not, *how* we live our life — including what we do and the type of person we choose to be — is a powerful *role model* that impacts the lives of others, especially children, grandchildren, siblings, and close friends.

So, for all the reasons cited above, several years ago I made the decision that for the rest of my life I would pursue non-overeating and weight control over overeating and weight non-control. I figured it would help me become the finest person I can be, create the most beneficial life I can create, and possibly help others do the same.

An Interesting Discovery

In the six-year span of creating, testing, and refining the Weight Success Method an interesting thing happened. I discovered that the amount of immediate pleasure and enjoyment derived from a particular good activity — in this case, right eating and weight control — isn't necessarily a fixed amount. I realized that the immediate enjoyment to be derived from right eating and weight control can be *expanded*. For some ways of doing that, go to the *Eight Actions for Easier Calorie Control* chapter (p. **102**).

Summing Up

Here in a nutshell is how healthy-weight enjoyment happens. I derive daily enjoyment and motivation from doing the five daily actions of the Weight Success Method because by doing these actions I experience enjoyment from (a) achieving and seeing daily personal progress, (b) delivering and receiving positive self-reinforcement, (c) triumphing over occasional adversity or setback, (d) being director of my eating, (e) daily focusing on an exciting ultimate goal, and (f) feeling like a winner by performing daily winning actions.

I also derive enjoyment and motivation from (g) succeeding at living in my healthy-weight range, which makes me feel like a high-achiever, (h) realizing exciting weight success benefits from living at my healthy weight, and (i) maintaining awareness of these benefits on a daily basis.

And, finally, I derive enjoyment and gratification from (j) the act of improving my self and my life by pursuing a productive activity in place of a counterproductive one, or by living in my healthy-weight range rather than outside it, and from (k) being a living example that achieving *easier* healthy-weight living is *doable*, thereby inspiring others to "give it a go."

So, the Weight Success Method is not only the easiest and most effective way to healthy-weight living, it's also probably the most enjoyable and gratifying.

> Easiest **+** Most Effective **+** Most Enjoyable & Gratifying **=** **Super Weight-management Tool**

> # One of the secrets to lifelong happiness is:
> Savor and mentally expand good pleasures, and ignore and avoid bad pleasures. *Good pleasures* are those pleasures that contribute to you becoming a finer person, creating a more beneficial life, and helping others do the same. *Bad pleasures* are those that detract from those three things. This applies to virtually every aspect of living, including relationships, work, recreation, exercise, <u>and</u> eating.

CHAPTER 18: Why the Weight Success Method Gets Your Whole Mind Involved

This chapter explains the interaction between the Weight Success Method and your mind. It could be eye-opening ... or, perhaps more correctly, mind-opening.

FOR THE PAST 50 years we've been seeking "the easy way to weight control." We've been expecting it to be some new-tech, new-pill, new-surgery, new-food, new-diet, new-exercise, new-gimmick thing. But no one has found it. One reason is, a main key to easier weight control isn't in the physical world; it's in the <u>mind</u> world. It's this: Have your *whole* mind — that is, both conscious <u>and</u> subconscious mind — involved each day in the pursuit of living in your healthy-weight range. This is a main driver of successful weight management. (For more on this, see the Whole Mind Involvement section (p. **28**) in the Success Drivers section of Chapter Two.)

Those who are succeeding at creating easier healthy-weight living are applying this dynamic — either knowingly or unknowingly, intentionally or non-intentionally. Those who are not yet succeeding at creating healthy-weight living are not yet applying this dynamic.

As previously stated, the easiest way to get both your conscious *and* subconscious mind involved in the daily pursuit of living in your healthy-weight range is apply the five daily actions of the Weight Success Method each day. I'm now going to explain why this is. It involves knowing how the mind — in particular, the subconscious mind — works.

How Your Mind Works: An Overview

Here's a "weird little thing" you may have not yet realized: The conception you hold of your own mind determines to a large extent the way your mind performs. Yes, it's true. So here's a conception that can lead to getting optimal performance and benefits from your mind.

View your mind as a two-part entity with each part possessing certain faculties and performing certain functions.

Further, view these two parts of your mind as working together as a team, with one part being the upfront member of the team, which we'll call *conscious mind,* and the other part being the behind-the-scenes member of the team, which we'll call *subconscious mind.* Further assume that you are a unique human being that possesses a certain unique spiritual identity, which we'll call *I* or *self.* Assume that this *I* or *self* identity resides mainly in the conscious part of your mind.

Further, assume that this conscious–subconscious mind team performs a certain set of team functions — that is, functions that the team members perform jointly.

Still further, assume that one of these team functions is a function that lies at the core of everything the team does. We'll call it *creation function.*

Further, assume that this creation function involves two processes: the first process being to identify creation opportunities and the second process being to actualize those creation opportunities that have been identified. Your conscious mind mainly works on the first process; your subconscious mind mainly works on the second one.

We'll call the first process *conceptualizing* and the second process *actualizing.* Each results in a certain type of outcome. The outcome of conceptualizing is conceptualizations, or *imagined situations.* The outcome of actualizing is actualizations, or *actual situations.*

So, a main role of your conscious mind is to identify imagined situations for actualizing and a main role of your subconscious mind is to actualize these imagined situations. Or, put more concisely, a main role of your subconscious mind is to *actualize the content of your conscious mind.*

Now here's a key point. Your subconscious mind strives to perform this actualizing role automatically and diligently. It goes at it 24/7, and you can't stop it, and it continues up to the moment you die.

Most people are unaware of the actualizing function and power of their subconscious mind. This is because this activity goes on "behind the scenes," or in a realm apart from the conscious mind. But, even though it may go largely unnoticed by most people, the actualizing action of your subconscious mind has been playing a major role in determining what you do each day of your life, including what and how much you eat.

Conscious Mind Content

So, a main function of your subconscious mind is to actualize the content of your conscious mind. This leads to a question: What is the "content" of your conscious mind? Simply put, the main content of your conscious mind is desires and perspectives.

I define *desire* as an imagined situation that you'd like to see become an actual situation. We apply various labels to our desires. Some of the most common are: goal, dream, plan, aspiration, hope, wish, and, of course, desire.

I define *perspective* as a mental view or depiction you hold about some aspect of your self, your mind, your life, or the world about you. We apply various labels to our perspectives. Some of the most common are: belief, assumption, conviction, conjecture, conception, attitude, outlook, viewpoint, and, of course, perspective. Also, an interpretation of something we believe happened in the past is a form of perspective, and an expectation of something we believe will happen in the future is a form of perspective.

How Your Subconscious Mind Actualizes

So, your subconscious mind strives 24/7 to actualize the dominant desires and perspectives, or dominant imagined situations, held in your conscious mind. This now leads to the next key question: How, exactly, does your subconscious mind actualize a particular desire or perspective (a.k.a. imagined situation) held in your conscious mind?

Answer: It does it through performing one or both of these two processes:

1 – It acts to *validate* the particular desire or perspective; and/or,

2 – It acts to *materialize* the particular desire or perspective.

To **validate** a particular desire or perspective your subconscious mind creates *thoughts* and *feelings* that align with, or corroborate, the desire or perspective.

To **materialize** a particular desire or perspective your subconscious mind creates *thoughts* and *feelings* that guide you to perform actions that lead to the creation of an actual situation that corresponds to the imagined situation (desire or perspective).

By one or both of these two processes your subconscious mind works to actualize, or "make real," any particular dominant desire or perspective (a.k.a. imagined situation) held in your conscious mind.

So, the way your subconscious mind brings about easier healthy-weight living is: When motivated to do so, it creates *thoughts* and *feelings* that steer you toward performing actions that lead to the actualization of healthy-weight living. Here are examples of how this can happen.

If, for example, you were to motivate your subconscious mind to assist you with doing more right eating and less wrong eating it would create thoughts and feelings that steer you toward right eating and away from wrong eating.

If you were to motivate it (your subconscious mind) to assist with surmounting a certain impediment to creating healthy-weight living, it would create thoughts and feelings that steer you toward sidestepping or surmounting that impediment. By the way, any fat-promoting factor, such as one of those cited in the Fat-promoting Factors list on page **20**, is a surmountable "impediment."

If you were to motivate it (your subconscious mind) to assist with finding a more effective dietary program it would create thoughts and feelings that steer you toward finding or contacting such a program.

If you were to motivate it to assist with acquiring some additional know-how or information it would create thoughts and feelings that steer you toward discovering a source that contains that know-how or information.

If you were to motivate it to assist with getting a certain type of input or assistance it would create thoughts and feelings that steer you toward finding or making contact with a person or program that specializes in providing such assistance.

If you were to motivate it to assist with helping you adopt a certain perspective necessary for expediting easier healthy-weight living, it would create thoughts and feelings that steer you toward a situation that results in you gaining that perspective.

And, finally, if you were to motivate your subconscious mind to assist with squelching a certain overeating habit and replacing it with a right-eating habit, it would create thoughts and feelings that assist with subduing the overeating habit and with installing the right-eating habit. (For more on habits, go to the Key to Beating the Bad Habit of Unguided Eating chapter, page **152**.)

To sum up, to create healthy-weight living more easily you must involve your WHOLE mind, including subconscious mind, in your pursuit of healthy-weight living. Once you do this your mind applies its *full* faculties to the process. And, when your mind's full faculties are at work, healthy-weight living happens and happens *easily,* or at least way more easily than you've likely ever thought possible. In short, the more involved your subconscious mind is in your pursuit of healthy-weight living, the easier the creation of healthy-weight living becomes.

Here's an infographic that sums up this discussion on how easier healthy-weight living happens.

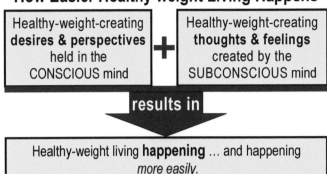

How Easier Healthy-weight Living Happens

Healthy-weight-creating **desires & perspectives** held in the CONSCIOUS mind **+** Healthy-weight-creating **thoughts & feelings** created by the SUBCONSCIOUS mind

results in

Healthy-weight living **happening** … and happening *more easily.*

So, in this section I've provided a general overview of how your mind works. Now I need to describe how your subconscious mind affects eating and weight management. For this I must add some specifics, which includes further insights into the subconscious mind and how it works.

A Perspective on the Subconscious Mind

A hundred years or so ago psychologists tended to depict the subconscious mind as a capricious, wild, inscrutable, infantile, non-directable "force." Since then other perspectives of it have emerged. Which raises the question: Of all the various perspectives of the subconscious mind, which one is the correct one? My answer: Perhaps each of them, *depending on the situation.*

How can that be? It's for this reason. My experience tells me that my subconscious mind will essentially perform in a manner consistent with the way I envision it performing. Meaning, whatever perspective I might hold of my subconscious mind, my subconscious mind pursues actualizing that perspective. This concept — if universally true, and I believe it is — carries significant ramification.

So, realizing that my subconscious mind strives to actualize, or make happen, the perspective I hold of it, I should be holding the following perspective. I view my subconscious mind as a responsive, reliable, helpful, directable, logical, creative, insightful, wise, dedicated partner perpetually committed to assisting me in becoming the finest person I can be and creating the most beneficial life I can create, and possessing vast powers and connections for answering the questions I pose to it and for actualizing the goals, directives, and expectations I submit to it. In short, I view it in the most positive, productive perspective possible. I urge you to view your subconscious mind in a similar way. I predict you'll be pleased — even amazed — by what happens.

How Your Subconscious Mind Determines What It Will Actualize

I just explained in general concept how you influence what the subconscious mind is and does. Now I explain it more specifically.

To decide on what it will actualize your subconscious mind takes cues from your conscious mind. These cues exist as two types: (1) deliberate communication sent from your conscious mind to your subconscious mind, and (2) observation by your subconscious mind of what your conscious mind is focusing on. I'll describe each.

Cue Type #1: DELIBERATE COMMUNICATION

Few people provide this type of cue to their subconscious mind. This is because few know about it. But sending deliberate communication to your subconscious mind is a powerful way to motivate it to do what you want it to be doing.

It's especially useful and effective when your subconscious mind has been spending years actualizing a particular undesirable situation, such as, for example, wrong eating, or overeating.

You can send deliberate communication to your subconscious mind three ways: by words, by images, by actions — otherwise called verbalization, visualization, and demonstration. Here's how each works.

Communication Way #1: Verbalization

Verbalization involves expressing a communication with words. It can be done either by speaking aloud, including in a whisper, or by "speaking silently in your mind." The five main types of verbalization messages are feedback, self-reinforce-

ment, directive, depiction, and feeling expression. I'll describe each.

Feedback. *Feedback* is information about past performance that enables us to achieve or maintain desired performance in the future. Along with being communicated verbally, feedback can also be expressed numerically and graphically. In the Weight Success Method timely feedback mainly derives from the daily weighing done in Daily Action 1 (p. **44**). It also can derive from any of the tools presented in Chapter 27 (p. **174**).

Self-reinforcement. When you convey appreciation and thanks to your self — or your mind — for having performed a certain desired action, or for having actualized a certain imagined desired situation, we call it *verbal self-reinforcement*. To add strength to the reinforcement we often include instructions to keep on doing the desired action. Our special label for this type of reinforcement communication is Thank You, Keep It Up message. A main example is the Thank You, Keep It Up message (p. **46**) used in Daily Action 2A. It's also used in the Guided Eating Process of Daily Action 5–Guided Eating (p. **56**).

Directive. When the communication takes the form of an instruction, order, or request conveyed to your subconscious mind we call it a *directive*. The Weight Success Method makes powerful use of directive-type communication. A main example is the Weight Success Benefits Directive used in Daily Action 3–Benefits Directive (p. **50**). Also, directive-type communication is used in the Guided Eating Process of Daily Action 5–Guided Eating.

Depiction. A *depiction* is a word description of a particular imagined situation. Typically it's of an imagined situation you want your subconscious mind to actualize (which it does by creating an actual situation that corresponds to the imagined situation). The Weight Success Method makes extensive powerful use of depiction statements. A main example is the Healthy-weight Goal Statement (p. **54**) described in Daily Action 4–Goal. It's also sometimes used in the Guided Eating Process of Daily Action 5.

Feeling Expression. When a verbalization conveys how you feel about a certain situation we call it a *feeling expression*. This type of communication tells your subconscious mind how you feel, or want to be feeling, about a situation. Feeling expressions that promote right eating and living in one's healthy-weight range occur within the five daily actions of the Weight Success Method.

Communication Way #2: Visualization

Visualization involves expressing a communication with images, or mental pictures. It comes in two forms: still image and moving image. A still image is a mental picture of a single situation or thing; basically a mental photograph. A moving image is a mental picture of a moving action or series of events; basically a mental movie or video. The mental movie can be in either third person or first person. In third person you're viewing yourself acting in the movie. In first person you're an actor in the process of making the movie. Some persons believe the first-person approach is more effective than the third-person.

Typically a visualization is of an imagined situation you want your subconscious mind to actualize, which it does by creating an actual situation that corresponds to the imagined situation. In the Weight Success Method you're sending a visualization communication to your subconscious mind every time you visualize the realization of one of your weight success benefits or visualize yourself being at your healthy weight.

Communication Way #3: Demonstration (or Acting As-if)

Demonstration — also called **acting as-if** — involves communicating with actions. The actions include both physical actions <u>and</u> mental actions. Precisely defined, acting as-if is the act of holding in mind an assumption that a particular situation presently exists or is in the process of coming about, *and then conducting your thinking, feelings, and actions in accordance with that assumption.* Put another way, it's doing a "real-life role-play" of a situation you want to exist or have happen.

Expressing a particular imagined situation via demonstration or acting as-if is a little known but very powerful means of communicating to your subconscious mind what you want it to be doing. It's used throughout the Weight Success Method.

Three Communication-enhancing Factors

Three factors determine the degree of impact your deliberate communications of cue type #1 have on motivating your subconscious mind to actualize a particular imagined situation. These three factors are: variety, frequency, and intensity. I'll describe each.

Variety. The more ways you communicate a particular imagined situation to your subconscious mind, the more diligently your subconscious mind works at actualizing the particular imagined situation. In doing the five daily actions of the Weight Success Method you use *all three* of the ways I just described — that is, verbalization, visualization, and demonstration or acting as-if.

Frequency. The more frequently you express a particular imagined situation to your subconscious mind, the more diligently your subconscious mind works at actualizing the particular imagined situation. In doing the five daily actions of the Weight Success Method you express certain imagined situations — mainly, right eating and healthy-weight living — *numerous* times throughout each day.

Lesser FREQUENCY of right-eating communication by the **conscious** mind — results in — lesser ASSISTANCE with creating right eating & healthy-weight living by the **subconscious** mind.	**&**	Greater FREQUENCY of right-eating communication by the **conscious** mind — results in — <u>greater</u> ASSISTANCE with creating right eating & healthy-weight living by the **subconscious** mind.

Intensity. The more intensely, or emotionally, you express a particular imagined situation to your subconscious mind, the more diligently your subconscious mind works at actualizing the particular imagined situation. When you do the five daily actions of the Weight Success Method you express certain healthy-weight-creating communications with emotional intensity at various times every day.

So to sum up, to maximize the impact of deliberate communication on motivating your subconscious mind to actualize a particular imagined situation — such as right eating and healthy-weight living — you do three things:

1. Communicate in *multiple* ways the imagined situation you want actualized;

2. Communicate *frequently* the imagined situation you want actualized;

3. Communicate with *emotional intensity* (at times) the imagined situation you want actualized.

What this means is: When you'd like your mind to diligently pursue actualizing a particular imagined situation or goal — such as the goal of living in your healthy-weight range the rest of your life — make this goal a highly important priority in the "eyes" of your subconscious mind. To do this, (a) communicate this priority to your subconscious mind in multiple ways, and (b) communicate it numerous times every day, and (c) at least some times every day communicate it with emotional intensity. Doing the five daily actions of the Weight Success Method each day results in you doing these three things as regards achieving the goal of healthy-weight living.

But, as powerful as deliberate communication is for directing one's subconscious mind, most persons never use it. So for these people how does their subconscious mind determine what it will actualize? It's by cue type #2.

Cue Type #2: CONSCIOUS MIND FOCUS

Although only a few people use cue type #1, cue type #2 operates with everyone. This cue consists of what the conscious mind regularly focuses on. It works like this.

There are hundreds of possible imagined situations your subconscious mind could pursue actualizing. But it will actualize only a few at a time.

That's because if it tried to pursue actualizing hundreds of imagined situations at the same time it would result in you being an ineffectual person living a confused, chaotic life.

So, how does your subconscious mind determine which imagined situations it will pursue actualizing? Answer: It strives to actualize those imagined situations that appear to it to be *most important* to you. And, how does it determine which imagined situations are most important to you? It observes what your conscious mind spends the *most time* focusing on — that is, thinking about, talking about, pursuing, and enjoyably doing. In short, as regards any particular imagined situation, *your subconscious mind assumes that greater amount of focus time means greater importance, and lesser amount means lesser importance.*

As a result, those imagined situations that receive the most amount of conscious mind focus time get the most "actualization effort" by your subconscious mind, and those situations that receive the least amount of conscious mind focus time get the least "actualization effort" by your subconscious mind. So how does this apply to the pursuit of healthy-weight living? It works like this.

Lesser FOCUS on right eating & healthy-weight living by the **conscious** mind — results in — lesser ASSISTANCE with creating right eating & healthy-weight living by the **subconscious** mind.	**&**	Greater FOCUS on right eating & healthy-weight living by the **conscious** mind — results in — greater ASSISTANCE with creating right eating & healthy-weight living by the **subconscious** mind.

What's more, if two imagined situations happen to be mutually exclusive — that is, only one can be actualized and not both — your subconscious mind will pursue actualizing the one that appears to it to be the most important of the two, and will ignore actualizing the other one. For example, right eating and wrong eating, or non-overeating and overeating, are mutually exclusive. So which one will your subconscious mind choose to actualize? *It will pursue actualizing the one that's receiving the greatest amount of conscious mind focus time, or is* being thought about, talked about, pursued, and enjoyed the greatest amount of time — and will ignore pursuing the opposing imagined situation.

All of which means, if you've been spending more time focusing on wrong eating than on right eating, your subconscious mind has been concluding that wrong eating is more important to you than right eating and, so, it has been focusing on actualizing wrong eating and ignoring actualizing right eating. Such a situation makes doing daily right eating nearly impossible, at least on a sustained basis, and makes doing daily wrong eating inevitable. This, by the way, explains why most folks are engaging in daily overeating.

It also explains why some are successful at losing weight but fail at keeping it off. While pursuing weight loss they have their conscious mind focusing intently each day on actualizing their weight-loss goal. But, once they achieve that goal they conclude that it's "job done" and, in doing so, they let their conscious mind cease its daily focus on weight management. This results in their subconscious mind ceasing to perform weight management activities. Which results in them failing to keep off the weight they lost. In short, they succeeded at weight loss because they focused daily on weight loss; they fail at weight maintenance because they *don't* focus daily on weight maintenance. (For more, go to The Secret Discovered section, page **20**.)

So, to summarize, if your conscious mind has been spending years focusing on wrong eating, your subconscious mind has been spending years concluding that wrong eating is what you want it to be actualizing, or bringing about. In such a situation, the easiest, quickest, most effective way to change your eating habits from wrong eating to right eating, or from overeating to non-overeating, is do two things:

1 – *Increase FOCUS.* Spend more conscious mind time focusing on right eating than on wrong eating — that is, spend more time thinking about, talking about, pursuing, and enjoyably doing right eating than wrong eating (this is cue type #2); and

2 – *Increase COMMUNICATION.* Send deliberate daily communications to your subconscious mind — specifically, communications that motivate it to (a) pursue right eating and avoid wrong eating and (b) pursue living in your healthy-weight range (cue type #1).

Or, in other words, use *both* cue types to motivate your subconscious mind to actualize your goal of easily engaging in right eating and living in your healthy-weight range.

Why the Five Daily Actions Work

One of the reasons the five daily actions of the Weight Success Method work and work easily is because these actions do two things: (1) they send *multiple kinds* of powerful healthy-weight-promoting communications *numerous times* each day to your subconscious mind, with some of these communications being delivered with *emotional* intensity and (2) they cause you to spend *more time* focusing on right eating than on wrong eating, and *more time* focusing on living in your healthy-weight range.

In the "eyes" of your subconscious mind, all this makes right eating to be more important than wrong eating, and makes living in your healthy-weight range to be very, *very* important. This, in turn, motivates your subconscious mind to actualize right eating and healthy-weight living for the rest of your life. And, by your subconscious mind doing this, healthy-weight living happens easily — or way more easily than you've ever imagined.

In short, by doing the Weight Success Method each day you each day involve your *whole* mind — that is, both conscious <u>and</u> subconscious mind — in the pursuit of living in your healthy-weight range. This results in your mind steering you away from overeating and toward non-overeating which, in turn, results in creating healthy-weight living for life. The infographic on the next page depicts "A Reason Why the Weight Success Method Works."

A Reason Why the Weight Success Method Works

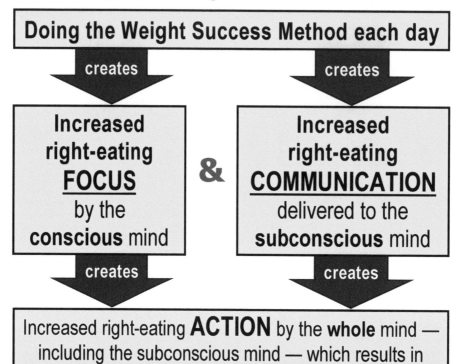

Right-eating FOCUS = Time spent thinking about, talking about, pursuing, and enjoyably doing right eating and healthy-weight living.

Right-eating COMMUNICATION = Communication that tells your subconscious mind to steer you toward right eating and healthy-weight living.

Three Concepts to Keep in Mind

1 – The more daily **focus** you put on right eating and healthy-weight living <u>and</u> the more right-eating **communication** you express, the more vigorously your mind — including subconscious mind — works at bringing about right eating and healthy-weight living.

2 – The more vigorously your subconscious mind works at bringing about right eating and healthy-weight living, the *easier* it becomes for you to achieve right eating and healthy-weight living.

3 – It doesn't matter how strong your overeating habits might be, there is a point at which a certain amount of right-eating **focus** and right-eating **communication** will result in your subconscious mind installing right-eating habits and urges that overwhelm and surmount the overeating habits and urges, and also surmount any fat-promoting factor that might apply to you or your life.

CHAPTER 19: Success Drivers and Success Killers in Depth

Doing the Weight Success Method installs success drivers into your weight success pursuit — and also diminishes success killers.

CHAPTER 2 described 19 vital elements (p. **23**) for succeeding at weight control and healthy-weight living. We dubbed them *success drivers*. This chapter 19 describes them in greater depth.

Success Driver **1:** ACHIEVEMENT GOAL

This driver involves identifying a desired ultimate outcome pertaining to a particular pursuit.

We call this desired ultimate outcome *achievement goal*. The vital function of an achievement goal is it provides an imagined desired situation that's held in the mind. When one holds an imagined desired situation (a.k.a. achievement goal) in mind it triggers one's mind, including one's subconscious mind, to create thoughts and feelings that guide one to perform actions that lead to achievement of the goal — or, in short, that lead to creation of an actual situation that corresponds to the imagined desired situation.

As pertains to your weight success pursuit, the Achievement Goal is: *To be the person of your healthy weight and be healthy, happy, and doing great.* (Note: Your *healthy weight* is every weight in your desired healthy-weight range.) We call this the Healthy-weight Goal.

> More on healthy-weight goal statement is described in *Daily Action 4* (p. **54**).

Success Driver **2:** FAILURE CAUSE AWARENESS

This driver involves recognizing the root activity or factor that causes setback — and perhaps failure — in a particular pursuit.

As pertains to the pursuit of weight control and healthy-weight living, the root activity causing failure is: *Overperformance* of a certain three-action process, the process of:

1 – Opening one's mouth;

2 – Inserting a piece of metabolizable calorie-containing food into one's mouth; and

3 – Swallowing the piece of food.

Overperformance of this process is the <u>real</u> cause and <u>only</u> cause of (a) weight gain and (b) weight control failure. And, it's *totally controllable* by each person. Recognizing this is the first step to succeeding at weight control and healthy-weight living. (More on failure cause awareness is described in *Startup Action 1,* page **35**.)

> **Note:** In this book the word *eating* encompasses drinking. And the word *food* encompasses beverages. So wherever you read the terms *eating* and *food* know that it includes drinking and beverages.

Success Driver **3:** GOAL-ACHIEVING MINDSET

This driver involves holding a mindset of goal-promoting views and beliefs, and acting as-if these views and beliefs are a true depiction of reality.

Along with working to actualize important goals, your mind — including subconscious mind — also works to actualize your dominant views and beliefs, especially those beliefs you *act on* each day, or act as-if are a true depiction of reality.

As pertains to your healthy-weight living Achievement Goal — there are two types of beliefs: goal-promoting and goal-hindering. Beliefs that steer you toward accomplishment of the goal we call *goal-promoting beliefs*. Beliefs that steer you away from goal accomplishment we call *goal-hindering beliefs*.

The more goal-promoting beliefs you hold in mind and act as-if are true the more your subconscious mind works at creating thoughts and feelings that steer you toward goal achievement.

> More on weight success mindset is described in *Startup Action 5* (p. **37**).

Mindset → Actions → Outcome

| Mindset | causes → | Actions | causes → | Outcome |

Success Driver **4**: ENJOYMENT OF PROCESS

This driver involves identifying or creating a process, or set of actions, by which daily enjoyment is derived from daily pursuit and progressive accomplishment of the Achievement Goal.

When you find the activity involved in achieving a goal to be fun, enjoyable, or otherwise gratifying to do, it makes it easier for you to accomplish the goal because you automatically put more time, focus, and energy into the process. So, as much as feasible you should strive to make the goal-achieving process of healthy-weight living to be fun, enjoyable, and/or gratifying. Yes, it *is* possible to do. To learn how, go to page **123.**

Success Driver **5**: MOTIVATING REASON

This driver involves identifying the main reason or reasons for pursuing the Achievement Goal.

As pertains to your weight success pursuit, the "main reasons" you have for doing it are the benefits you gain from living in your healthy-weight range. We call these benefits *weight success benefits*. The more clearly and frequently you envision them, the more good reason you have for striving to achieve lifelong weight success. Which, in turn, translates into greater daily motivation for living in your healthy-weight range.

> More on weight success benefits is described in *Startup Action 3* (p. **36**) and in the *Weight Success Benefits in Detail* chapter (p. **80**).

Success Driver **6**: MANDATE DECISION

This driver involves deciding that accomplishment of the Achievement Goal is a *mandatory* feature of one's life.

As pertains to your weight success pursuit, you must make the firm decision that living at your healthy weight is a <u>non</u>-optional, <u>will</u>-do, <u>must</u>-have aspect of your existence. You must make this

decision and commit to realizing it. Why? Because, if you don't you'll almost certainly fail at creating healthy-weight living.

Success Driver **7**: FEEDBACK SYSTEM

This driver involves identifying or creating a way of measuring daily performance pertaining to realization of the Achievement Goal.

As pertains to your weight success pursuit, the most powerful daily feedback system you can employ is: *daily weighing with an accurate bathroom scale.*

What do you do with this daily feedback? When the daily weight reading is a *desired* reading you deliver positive reinforcement to your self — that is, to your mind. When the reading is an *undesired* reading you respond by taking immediate corrective action.

An accurate daily weighing system that's *properly* used <u>each</u> day is the <u>most</u> powerful healthy-weight creation tool there is.

> More on feedback, reinforcement, and correction is described in *Daily Action 1* (p. **44**), *Daily Action 2A* (p. **45**), and *Daily Action 2B* (p. **48**).

Success Driver **8**: REMINDER SYSTEM

This driver involves installing a failproof reminder system.

As pertains to your weight success pursuit, this is a system that never fails to remind you each day to apply your preferred dietary program and daily action plan. This is critical for healthy-weight living success. Why? Because, failure to *remember* to do what one should be doing is a major cause of project failure.

> More on failproof reminder system is described in *Startup Action 8* (p. **41**).

Success Driver **9**: GOAL-ACHIEVING KNOWLEDGE

This driver involves acquiring knowledge vital to achievement of the Achievement Goal.

As pertains to creating weight success, the main goal-achieving knowledge you'll need for doing that is contained in this book. So, the way you acquire vital goal-achieving knowledge for healthy-weight living is: Read this book, especially Chapter 2.

Also, depending on the Preferred Dietary Prgram that you select, you might find it helpful to familiarize yourself with any special information pertaining to that program.

Success Driver 10: ESSENTIAL SUCCESS ACTIONS

This driver involves making sure that the essential success actions are done each day.

Some success actions are "helpful to do." Others are "critical to do every day" — meaning, if they're not done, the likelihood of achieving the Achievement Goal is greatly diminished. We call them *essential success actions*. It's imperative that you do the essential success actions every day.

What are the essential success actions in your weight success journey? They're Daily Actions 1–5 of the Weight Success Method (p. 44).

Doing essential success actions performs two vital functions. First, it maintains your *daily focus and motivation*. Second, it creates ongoing *daily progress* toward goal achievement. It's worth noting that doing essential success actions each day is at the core of virtually every successful significant personal pursuit.

So, *every day* for the rest of your life do the essential success actions aimed at achieving the goal of lifelong healthy-weight living. This is one of the ultimate keys to succeeding at creating lifelong weight success. Doing the Weight Success Method *makes this happen*.

Success Driver 11: DESIRE

This driver involves holding strong daily desire for realizing the Achievement Goal.

It also involves each day fueling this desire by calling to mind the reason for (or benefits to be derived from) goal achievement. Typically, the bigger the goal, the more desire is needed for accomplishing it.

Other terms for "desire" are passion, eagerness, determination.

As pertains to your weight success pursuit, this means if you want to succeed at realizing your Healthy-weight Goal, you need to hold *strong daily desire* for its accomplishment. If you don't you'll likely drift away from pursuing the goal and end up quitting. So, how do you hold strong daily desire for achieving your healthy-weight goal? You do these three things.

Firstly, you decide that achieving your healthy-weight goal is a *mandatory* feature of your existence.

Secondly, you hold the assumption — and also act as-if — achieving the goal is doable (and perhaps even *easily* doable).

Thirdly, each day you call to mind the *benefits* of goal achievement, and you visualize how good your life will be with these benefits. And, you hold the belief that these benefits are in the process of coming about each day.

The more times you think about, or visualize, the benefits of accomplishing your healthy-weight goal, the more you fuel your daily desire to achieve the goal. And, the stronger your daily desire is, the more your mind — including subconscious mind — assists with goal realization by creating thoughts and feelings that steer you toward that realization. In your weight success journey, we call these benefits *weight success benefits*.

More on weight success benefits is described in the *Weight Success Benefits in Detail* chapter (p. **80**).

Success Driver 12: FOCUS

This driver involves each day focusing on the Achievement Goal.

Or, put another way, it involves each day thinking about, talking about, pursuing, and/or deriving enjoyment from the accomplishment or progressive realization of the goal.

The more time you spend focusing on, or paying attention to, a particular goal, the more importance your subconscious mind attaches to that goal. And, the more importance your subconscious mind attaches to the goal, the more it acts to create thoughts and feelings that steer you toward accomplishment of the goal.

So, as pertains to your weight success journey, you must spend time each day *focusing* on the ongoing realization of your healthy-weight goal. A main purpose of doing the Weight Success Method is to cause this daily focusing to happen.

For more on focus, go to the "Cue Type #2: Conscious Mind Focus" section, p. **134**.

Success Driver **13**: SELF-COMMUNICATION

This driver involves sending goal-promoting communications to one's self each day.

Communications you send to your self we call *self-communications*. They are communications you send to your mind — including your subconscious mind. These communications describe what you want your mind to be doing in way of achieving a particular goal. Self-communications are delivered three ways: verbalization, visualization, and demonstration or acting as-if.

Goal-actualizing self-communications trigger your subconscious mind to create thoughts and feelings that make goal realization happen, or happen more easily. The more goal-actualizing self-communication you send, the more you motivate your mind — including subconscious mind — to assist with goal achievement.

If you'd like to read more discussion on this, go to the *Why the Weight Success Method Gets Your Whole Mind Involved* chapter, page **129**.

As pertains to your weight success pursuit, goal-promoting communications trigger your subconscious mind to create thoughts and feelings that make healthy-weight living happen more easily. The more goal-promoting communication you send, the more you motivate your subconscious mind to assist.

For more on self-communication, go to the "Cue Type #1: Deliberate Communication" section, p. **132**.

Success Driver **14**: PROGRESS TRACKING AND RESPONSE

This driver involves tracking one's daily performance and providing immediate positive response.

For tracking progress one needs feedback. *Feedback* is information that depicts past performance. When the feedback depicts *desired* past performance — a.k.a. progress — you deliver immediate self-reinforcement. When the feedback depicts *undesired* past performance you initiate immediate corrective action. Each is a positive response that expedites goal achievement. Also, for progress tracking to be optimally useful it must be timely. Meaning, for example, daily progress tracking (a.k.a. daily feedback) is usually more useful than, say, weekly progress tracking. In your weight success pursuit, the weight number you get from Daily Action 1 (daily weighing) is the most useful tracking feedback in your weight success journey.

For other examples of progress measuring tools, go to the *Handy Extra Tools* chapter (p. **174**).

Success Driver **15**: SELF-REINFORCEMENT

This driver involves delivering reinforcement — such as appreciation and praise — to one's self after daily progress happens, and telling oneself to keep up the good work.

What is reinforcement? The act of giving someone something they like as a response or consequence for performing a certain action or creating a certain result is known as *reinforcement* — a.k.a. positive reinforcement. When that "someone" is our self, or our mind, we call it *self-reinforcement*.

When you deliver self-reinforcement, or appreciation and praise, to your mind — in particular, to your subconscious mind — after it provides assistance with creating a certain desired performance or result, it motivates your mind to continue providing that assistance in the future. In short, desired performance plus reinforcement creates more desired performance. (More on reinforcement is described in *Daily Action 2A*, page **45**.)

Success Driver **16:** SETBACK SURMOUNTING

This driver involves holding a productive perspective whenever there's a setback, and also enacting immediate corrective action and converting the setback into a progress action.

In every major endeavor — including the pursuit of weight success — setbacks occur. Success depends on the response to these setbacks. When one responds in a counterproductive way it results in turmoil, frustration, and defeat. But when one responds in a productive way it results in (a) learning from the setback and (b) converting it into a progress action.

> More on setback surmounting is described in *Daily Action 2B* (p. **48**) and also in the *Setback Reversal Made Easier* chapter (p. **88**).

Success Driver **17:** PERSISTENCE

This driver involves persistently pursuing the Achievement Goal, and pressing on in spite of challenges, setbacks, or discouragement.

The realization that unceasing persistence is a key to achieving any major goal isn't new; it has been around for decades. Many names have been applied to it. Examples include: persistence, perseverance, determination, tenacity, doggedness, pressing on, stick-to-it-ness, gutting-it-out, and grit.

So, as pertains to your weight success journey, *don't give up*. Instead, each day press on toward accomplishment of your worthy healthy-weight goal. If you do this, along with doing the Weight Success Method, you *will* achieve your goal.

Success Driver **18:** GOAL-ACHIEVING RELATIONSHIPS

This driver involves discovering and building relationships that encourage and assist one in accomplishing the Achievement Goal.

This success driver does not apply to every type of pursuit. But it can be made to apply to most. And, when it is applied it can be powerful.

As pertains to your weight success pursuit, productive relationships can expedite realization of your healthy-weight goal at least two ways. First, they can be a means for sustaining motivation and productive mindset during the pursuit of the goal. Second, they can be a means for obtaining valuable assistance — such as, advice, know-how, key resources — that can be helpful in expediting goal achievement. This assistance can be obtained from productive interaction with people and also God.

Lastly, it's important to note that one might find it helpful to downplay relationships or interactions that run counter to achievement of one's life-enhancing goals.

> For more on relationships, see the *Escaping Schadenfreude* chapter (p. **121**) and the relationships section (p. **160**) of the *How the Weight Success Method Enhances Your Life Journey* chapter, and the *Three Steps to Getting Input from God* section (p. **117**).

Success Driver **19:** WHOLE-MIND INVOLVEMENT

This driver involves having one's whole mind — that is, both conscious <u>and</u> subconscious mind — involved each day in the pursuit of the Achievement Goal.

As pertains to your weight success pursuit, when your whole mind is involved each day in the pursuit of your healthy-weight goal something powerful happens. It results in your subconscious mind stepping up and assisting with the achievement of that goal. Your subconscious mind does this by creating thoughts and feelings that make you more effective at (a) surmounting obstacles and (b) obtaining what you need for goal achievement. Which means, the more involved your subconscious mind is in the achievement of your healthy-weight goal, the easier the achievement of that goal becomes.

When your subconscious mind is working to steer you toward living in your healthy-weight range it creates healthy-weight-promoting thoughts and feelings that guide you toward healthy-weight living. This results in you doing right eating and weight control. Conversely, when your subconscious mind *isn't* involved in steering you toward living in your healthy-weight range it *doesn't* create healthy-weight-promoting thoughts and feelings. This results in overeating and weight gain. And, when you cycle between the two — that is, your subconscious mind is involved for a period, stops being involved for a period, starts again, stops again — you lose weight, gain weight, lose weight, gain weight — a condition called yo-yo dieting.

I call all that *The Whole-mind Dynamic of Healthy-weight Living*. Most people are unaware of this dynamic. So, they don't realize that a main success driver of healthy-weight living is:

> Have your WHOLE mind — that is, both conscious <u>and</u> subconscious mind — involved *each day* in the pursuit of living in your healthy-weight range.

As an infographic the Whole-mind Dynamic looks like this.

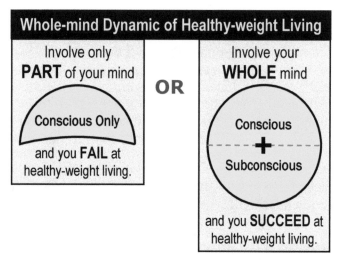

So, be sure to include this Success Driver 19 in your weight success journey.

Does the thought of "having your whole mind involved each day in the pursuit of living in your healthy-weight range" seem complex or hard to do? Well, good news, it's not. It's actually simple and easy **if** you do this: <u>Apply the Weight Success Method</u>. Doing the five daily actions of the Weight Success Method (p. 44) typically takes less than eight minutes a day. Yet it causes you to have your WHOLE mind involved *each day* in the pursuit of healthy-weight living. And this, in turn, *greatly* increases the likelihood of you succeeding at creating healthy-weight living for life.

For more on whole mind involvement, go to the *Why the Weight Success Method Gets Your Whole Mind Involved* chapter (p. **129**).

Societal Impact of the Whole Mind Dynamic

Here's how the Whole-mind Dynamic applies society-wide. Those few people who are living in their healthy-weight range likely have their *whole* mind — or both conscious <u>and</u> subconscious mind — involved each day in the pursuit of healthy-weight living. This involvement of their whole mind comes about either intentionally or non-intentionally or both.

Conversely, most of those people who are continuing to live <u>above</u> their healthy-weight range do *not* have their whole mind involved each day in the pursuit of healthy-weight living.

What's more, those who lost weight *while* dieting and then gained the weight back *after* the dieting had their whole mind involved *during* the dieting but stopped having their whole mind involved *after* the dieting!

Trying to achieve your biggest goals using only the "conscious half" of your mind is like trying to take a canoe trip using "half a canoe." Applying the Weight Success Method is the easiest way to ensure you're taking your whole canoe on your weight success journey.

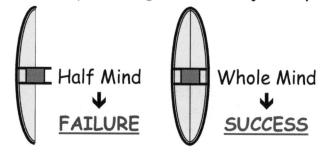

21 Success Killers

This section examines the flip-side of the weight success coin. It describes 21 activities that can cause a person to fail at weight control and healthy-weight living or, at least, cause the person to experience needless hassle and difficulty in achieving weight control. We dub these 21 activities *success killers*.

Put simply, the easiest, most effective way to succeed at healthy-weight living is this: (a) *include* as many success drivers as you can and (b) *exclude* or avoid as many success killers as you can. Doing this expands to the max the likelihood of creating lifelong healthy-weight living.

You'll note that many of these success killers are an "opposite action" to a success driver. So, doing the particular success driver automatically eliminates the opposing success killer.

Here are the 21 success killers you should strive to avoid:

1 – Believing that there's "no problem" in being "a little bit" overweight. ✎ This success killer causes one to do nothing when only slightly overweight. This is a problem, because being slightly overweight usually is the first step to becoming *a lot* overweight. So avoid this success killer by eliminating overweightness in any amount.

2 – Believing that there are factors beyond one's control that are making one overeat and gain weight. Or, put another way, it's holding the belief that weight control is impossible. ✎ This success killer causes one to avoid pursuing weight control because it promotes the rationalization that no matter what one does there are uncontrollable factors that will make one fail at weight control. So avoid this success killer by realizing that you have full control of your healthy-weight living destiny. (For the real cause of weight gain, see Success Driver 2, page **137**.)

3 – Believing that weight control is hard to do. ✎ This factor isn't as harmful as #2, but it's still a weight control saboteur. It causes one to

procrastinate on weight control because humans shun hardship, at least as involves eating. Plus it's self-fulfilling. When we believe something will be hard to do our mind often ensures that it is. How so? It's because our subconscious mind automatically creates thoughts, feelings, and actions that actualize our dominant views and beliefs. So avoid this success killer by realizing that most likely weight control is easier than you ever imagined it could be.

4 – Believing that doing weight control is unpleasant and enjoyment-robbing. ✎ Weight control requires making changes, and change is often unpleasant, especially when it involves giving up a daily pleasure. This causes one to procrastinate on weight control because most of us don't like losing a daily pleasure. So avoid this success killer by realizing that weight control can actually be pleasurable and enjoyable.

> Truth is, when done the right way, weight control and healthy-weight living creates *more* enjoyment than is lost — meaning, it can be an enjoyment *builder.* For more on this, see the *Why the Weight Success Method is Enjoyable* chapter (p. **123**) and also the Right Eating section in Startup Action 6 (p. **39**).

5 – Believing that lack of exercise causes overweightness and that more exercise is a requirement for creating weight control and weight success. ✎ This success killer causes one to fail at weight control because it blinds one to the real cause of weight gain (for that, see Success Driver 2, page **137**). So avoid this success killer by realizing that even though exercise is a beneficial activity a lack of exercise is not the cause of overweightness and more exercise is not the guaranteed cure.

> One of the biggest false assumptions of our society is that weight gain and overweightness is a result of too little exercise. This is a myth. Weight gain can occur even with a lot of exercise. Conversely, weight control and healthy-weight living can happen even with no exercise.

6 – Not realizing that the first step to weight-control success is *mindset* change. ✎ Overweightness is a physical condition. But the first step to conquering overweightness doesn't involve taking a physical action. Rather, it involves taking a *mental* action, or making a change in one's mindset — that is, a change in one's views and beliefs regarding eating and weight control. Without this first step, lifelong weight control and healthy-weight living usually don't happen. So avoid this success killer by making one of your first steps be the adoption of a healthy-weight-promoting mindset. (For more on this, see Startup Action 5, page **37**.)

7 — Not identifying one's desired healthy-weight range. Or, put another way, it's using a single weight number as one's target, or goal. ✎ Here's how this success killer undermines weight control. By having a single weight number as one's target, or goal, it makes one be a weight management loser on many days. This, in turn, tends to make one quit the pursuit of weight control. To enable yourself to be a weight management winner on most days, define a reasonable weight *range* as your goal. (For more on this, see Startup Action 2, page **36**.)

8 — Not deciding that healthy-weight living is *mandatory*. ✎ If you don't make the firm decision that healthy-weight living is a <u>non</u>-optional, <u>will</u>-do, <u>must</u>-have aspect of your existence, you will give up and quit as soon as the first inevitable little setback or discouragement arises. So avoid this success killer by deciding that healthy-weight living is a *mandatory* feature of your existence. (For more on this, see Startup Action 4, page **36**.)

9 — Not identifying one's weight success benefits. ✎ If you don't have strong, ample reason for pursuing weight control and healthy-weight living, you will lack full motivation for pursuing it. And, lacking full motivation will result in less than full results. So avoid this success killer by identifying all your weight success benefits. (For more on this, see Startup Action 3, page **36**, and also the Weight Success Benefits in Detail chapter, p. **80**.)

10 — Not identifying healthy-weight calorie consumption as the top priority of eating. ✎ There are two mutually exclusive top priorities in eating: (1) eating pleasure maximiza-tion and (2) healthy-weight calorie consumption. The first priority leads to overeating and weight gain. The second leads to non-overeating and healthy-weight living. To succeed at creating lifelong healthy-weight living one must embrace healthy-weight calorie consumption as the top priority. So avoid this success killer by adopting healthy-weight calorie consumption as your foremost eating priority. (For more on this, see Startup Action 6, page **39**.)

11 — Not adopting a dietary program that fits *you*. ✎ To achieve optimal success at weight control and healthy-weight living, most persons must apply a preferred dietary program. Further, this program must be applied fully. Finally, the easiest dietary program to apply fully is one that fits *you*, or that best fits your personal needs, desires, and lifestyle. So avoid this success killer by adopting a dietary program that best fits *you*. (For more on this, see Startup Action 7, page **40**.)

12 — Not remembering to do what one needs to be doing every day. ✎ You can have the best daily action plan in the world. But if you often fail to remember to apply it, all is lost. So, as pertains to your healthy-weight living daily action plan (which is the Weight Success Method), you need to have a failproof reminder mechanism that guarantees that you remember to do the Method each day. So avoid this success killer by installing a failproof reminder mechanism. (For more on this, see Startup Action 8, page **41**.)

13 — Not getting daily feedback derived from daily weighing. ✎ Without having *daily* feedback on one's body weight one lacks information for dispensing daily self-reinforcement and for taking daily corrective action when needed. And, without daily self-reinforcement and corrective action, one's weight control and healthy-weight living effectiveness suffers. So avoid this success killer by correctly weighing yourself *every* day. (For more on daily weighing, see Daily Action 1, page **44**.)

14 — Not keeping healthy-weight living a *top* priority. ✎ To succeed at any significant pursuit — including healthy-weight living — achieving success at the pursuit must be a top priority. If it's not, your mind — including subconscious mind — won't vigorously contribute the thoughts and feelings needed for creating that success. So avoid this success killer by holding healthy-weight living as a top priority in your life.

15 – Not responding to setbacks in a productive way. ✐ In every major pursuit, including the pursuit of healthy-weight living, setbacks happen. When one fails to respond productively to setbacks something bad happens. Discouragement and continued bad performance set in, and eventually one quits. So avoid this success killer by responding productively to every setback. (For more on this, see Daily Action 2B, page **48**.)

16 – Not ignoring negative comments by others. ✐ Receiving negative, discouraging comment from others — especially those close to you — can be a demotivator and major drag on one's weight control efforts. So, if you should be the target of such comment, do your best to ignore it. (For more on this, see the Escaping Schadenfreude chapter, page **121**.)

17 – Not doing guided eating most of the time. Or, put another way, doing _unguided_ eating most of the time. ✐ In terms of control, there are two types of eating: unguided and guided. Unguided eating leads to overeating and weight gain. Guided eating leads to weight control and healthy-weight living. To avoid unguided eating apply the Guided Eating Process described in Daily Action 5 (p. **56**).

18 – Not viewing healthy-weight maintenance as a noteworthy achievement. ✐ As a people, we applaud persons for the amount of weight they lose; then say nothing when they succeed at keeping the lost weight off. This reaction is cockeyed. Even though losing weight is commendable, _maintaining_ one's desired healthy weight is the truly exceptional accomplishment. When you fail to

view it that way, you rob yourself of deserved joy and motivation. So avoid this success killer by deriving a good feeling each day from your noteworthy accomplishment of continuing to live in your healthy-weight range. (For more on this, see The No-change Secret of Maintenance Achievement chapter, page **166**.)

19 – Not involving one's whole mind each day. ✐ When your whole mind — or both conscious <u>and</u> subconscious mind — is involved each day in the pursuit of healthy-weight living it results in your subconscious mind creating thoughts and feelings that guide you toward achievement of that goal. Conversely, when your subconscious mind _isn't_ involved it results in you being less-than-fully effective at creating healthy-weight living. So avoid this success killer by having your whole mind involved in your weight success pursuit. (For more on this, see Success Driver 19, page **141**.)

20 – Not applying a _daily_ success methodology for pursuing healthy-weight living. ✐ Applying a properly-constructed success methodology — a.k.a. daily success action plan — is one of the key tools for succeeding in any major personal pursuit. So avoid this success killer by applying a daily success methodology in your weight success pursuit. Tip: The easiest, most effective success methodology I know for pursuing healthy-weight living is the Weight Success Method, described in Chapter 2 (p. **19**).

21 – Not doing Weight Success Actions _every_ day, or not making each day be a Weight Success Day. ✐ When you don't pursue weight control and healthy-weight living as an ongoing daily success process — that is, as an ongoing process of doing vital Weight Success Actions each day — you eventually fail at healthy-weight living. So avoid this success killer by doing the Weight Success Method each day for the rest of your life. It typically takes _less than_ **8** minutes of dedicated time per day.

CHAPTER 20: 16 False Assumptions that Are Sabotaging Us

When it comes to weight management, it's <u>US</u> versus a World of False Assumptions, Delusions, and Wrong-headed Thinking.

THE WORLD abounds in false assumptions and misguided thinking pertaining to eating, weight gain, and weight management. This is one of the biggest obstacles we have to conquering over-weightness. Eradicating and circumventing these false assumptions is an essential step to creating nationwide healthy-weight living.

Within our society there exists 16 such assumptions that have been sabotaging our individual and national efforts at creating healthy-weight living and weight success. But we can break free of these beasts. Taking the approach of the Weight Success Method helps us identify these assumptions for what they are: harmful *false* beliefs.

So here are 16 false assumptions within our society that have been sabotaging our healthy-weight living and weight success efforts.

False Assumption 1: *Certain factors beyond individual control are causing us to overeat and be overweight.* ❧ There's an insidious trend afoot. This trend is spawning a crazy delusion that's sabotaging our efforts to conquer overweightness and create healthy-weight living. The trend I'm referring to is the "movement to discover factors that cause overeating and fat gain." I call these factors *fat-promoting factors*. Here are some that, so far, have been cited as things that are "causing" overeating and fat gain: genes, hormones, heredity, body chemistry, brain function, gender, age, menopause, lifestyle, too slow rate of metabolism, expanded appetite or food cravings, decreased smoking, anxiety, stress, depression, lack of sleep, lack of fiber, lack of fatty acids, eating at the wrong time, skipping breakfast, eating foods in the wrong sequence, eating too fast, eating foods derived from grains, eating foods containing "hidden carbs," low-fat foods, salt, sugar, artificial sweeteners, potato chips, food advertising, fast-food restaurants, availability of packaged foods made with too much sugar, artificial additives in food, low cost of food

due to agricultural innovation, taste buds insensitivity, too little exercise, working night shifts, unhealthy friends and family, glamorization of overweightness, criticism of overweightness, hearing people talk about body weight, thinking you're overweight, too many plus-sized models, yo-yo dieting, age and weight of your mother when you were born, level of carbon monoxide in the atmosphere, indoor temperature too high, lack of air conditioning during hot months, living near a noisy highway or railway or airline flight path, doing repeated decision-making at work, environmental factors that promote eating, endocrine disrupting chemicals such as bisphenol A and phthalates, environmental chemicals such as flame retardants, types of bacteria in your intestine, increasing abundance of food in modern society, certain viruses such as adenoviruses, and certain drugs such as medications that treat depression, heartburn, diabetes, inflammation, allergies, hypothyroidism, hypertension, contraception, and mental illness. Yes, every one has been cited as a factor causing overeating or overweightness.

And, amazingly, the list keeps growing! The above array of fat-promoting factors is current as of *December 2015*. It's much larger as of the date you're reading this, because since 2015 the obsessive quest to "discover" new scapegoat fat-promoting factors has been surging onward.

Not surprisingly, this "science of fat-promoting factors" is super-seductive. When I first encountered it it seemed like some of these factors pertained to me. It seemed like they might be the cause of my overeating and weight gain. Finally, I realized that this "discovering fat-promoting factors craze" is creating one of the craziest, most harmful national delusions in history. It's the *"I can't control my weight"* delusion. This is a *very* dangerous thing. It's dangerous because it leads to the copout conclusion "There's no point in me even trying."

Don't be sucked into the growing fat-promoting factors movement. Don't let the media hype that publicizes it make you believe you don't control your destiny when it comes to healthy-weight living. Because, you *do* control it.

Sure, some of these fat-promoting factors might promote overeating and make it easier to gain weight. But not a one *causes* a person to overeat or be overweight. Overeating and overweightness are caused by one thing only: overperformance of a certain 3-action process, the process of opening our mouth, inserting food into our mouth, and swallowing the food — a process that happens to be *totally controllable* by each of us. Our failure to recognize and act on this truth is a main factor preventing our creating healthy-weight living. And, this false assumption #1 is a main factor that's causing us to not act on that truth.

False Assumption 2: *If you're only slightly overweight it's okay because there are no bad consequences to it.* ✍ This is a self-comforting myth. Yes, it's true that being only slightly overweight is not as harmful as being greatly overweight. <u>But</u>, any degree of overweightness is still a problem, if for no other reason than this: Being slightly overweight seldom stays that way. It almost always leads to *greater* overweightness, or, at the least, to a lifetime of endless yo-yo dieting.

False Assumption 3: *Most humans lack the capability to control how much they eat.* ✍ This insidious assumption drives much of what's happening in today's world of weight control. Much of what's being proposed and pushed by government, corporations, and health organizations is based on this assumption. But, because it's inherently offensive it's seldom articulated; it's implicit, not explicit.

And, why is it offensive? Because if it were true, we'd no longer be human beings; we'd be something other than human. Worms, fish, pigs, dogs, and every other animal lacks the capability to deliberately determine how much it should eat. They eat by instinct or inborn behavior. But humans possess the capability to determine and control how much they eat. It comes with "being human." So, we should squelch the unarticulated implicit assumption that we lack this capability, otherwise folks might eventually start believing it ... and then start *acting as-if it's true.*

False Assumption 4: *Healthy-weight eating, or right eating, is hard to do.* ✍ This assumption is one of the great deterrents to people striving for healthy-weight living. They believe eating right foods in the right amount has just got to be painful and difficult. So they procrastinate on pursuing healthy-weight living. Fact is, healthy-weight eating is <u>not</u> hard to do. Or, if you prefer, it doesn't have to be hard to do. It all depends on what one believes and desires. When a person believes it will be easy to do, and strongly desires for it to be that way, they can and will find a way to make it that way.

False Assumption 5: *Healthy-weight eating is a pleasure-lacking, enjoyment-robbing experience.* ✍ As with Assumption 4, this assumption is also a deterrent to striving for healthy-weight living. But, healthy-weight eating, or right eating, doesn't have to be pleasure-lacking and enjoyment-robbing. It depends on what one believes and desires. When a person believes that healthy-weight eating can and will be enjoyable, and strongly desires for it to be that way, they can and will find a way to make it that way. Perhaps what we need is a new style of cuisine, a cuisine dedicated to creating foods that promote right eating — in other words, a *right-eating cuisine.*

False Assumption 6: *The main priority of eating is — or should be — pleasure maximization.* ✍ This assumption is one of the most pernicious. Why? Because, when a person's <u>main</u> eating priority, goal, or focus is pleasure maximization, their eating always extends into *overeating* — if not all the time at least enough of the time to create ongoing weight gain. This assumption is a stealthy manipulator that makes overeating *inevitable.*

It's also one of the hardest to debunk. This is because it's widespread and deeply entrenched in our society. So most people unquestionably accept it as fact. And, when you suggest that it's not the best way to approach eating, for the reason cited above, they tend to launch a host of defense mechanisms. Not least of which is trying to turn the suggestion into a joke. So, what's the best way to approach eating? It's to make your main eating priority to be healthy-weight calorie consumption. This involves the three priorities of *right eating*. (For more this, go to page **39** in Startup Action 6.)

False Assumption 7: *The main key to weight-control success is to find the right diet program.* Many people hold the belief that the key to their creating healthy-weight living lies in finding that one perfect diet program that works best. And, they further hold the belief that without finding such a program they're doomed to failure. So they spend years searching for the perfect program. But, ultimately, they never find a program that works for them. Why is that?

It's because, what makes any bona fide diet program work *isn't* the program, per se. Rather, it's whether or not the program is *fully* applied.

When a person applies a bona fide diet program fully, or the way it's intended to be applied, it usually works. When a person doesn't apply a program fully, it usually doesn't work, or works only partially. In short, partial application creates partial or no results; full application creates full results. So, we would be better served to spend less time focusing on the "which diet program is best" question and more time on the "how do we motivate our self to fully apply the dietary program of our choice" question.

Now, to ensure I'm not being misinterpreted, I point out that some diet programs are a better fit for you and your situation than are other programs. And, these "better fitting" programs are easier for you to fully apply. So they're the programs you might want to focus on. But, again, any bona fide diet program that's applied fully typically works fully and any that's not applied fully typically doesn't work fully. And, now, a reminder question: What's the easiest way to motivate yourself to do a diet program fully? Do the Weight Success Method.

False Assumption 8: *Lack of exercise is the cause of overweightness and more exercise is the solution.* Certainly, regular exercise is helpful and good. And every person would be well advised to do it. But, the belief that lack of exercise is the cause of overweightness and more exercise is the solution is erroneous and sometimes self-defeating. It can be self-defeating because *overweightness is caused by overeating, not by under-exercising!* What makes this Assumption 8 so harmful is it diverts people's attention from the real cause of overweightness: eating too much. This dooms many persons to years of frenetic exercising while still gaining weight — a discouraging situation, indeed. In short, exercise doesn't replace right eating, at least not in the long run; but it can work well as a complement to it.

False Assumption 9: *Weighing yourself each day is counterproductive, so avoid it.* This is one of the most misguided myths of the weight management world. Yes, daily weighing can be counterproductive when it's done the wrong way. But, virtually every activity in life is counterproductive when done the wrong way. Daily Action 1 (p. **44**) describes the right way. Do it the right way and daily weighing becomes one of the most powerful tools there is for conquering weight gain and creating healthy-weight living.

False Assumption 10: *Food advertising causes people to eat more, so if we reduce food advertising we'll reduce people's overeating.* Decades ago we outlawed certain types of cigarette and liquor advertising. Did that put an end to smoking, drinking, and over-drinking? Obviously not. So why are some folks suggesting that the way to curb overeating and weight gain is to limit food and restaurant advertising?

Truth is, blaming business advertising is a red herring that obfuscates what really needs to be done to achieve nationwide healthy-weight living. It's government leaders blaming businesses for our weight failure situation when, in fact, the blame — if any is to be ascribed — should rest on the government leaders who have thus far failed to create a national program designed to motivate and equip people to voluntarily engage in right eating. Having such a program would actually result in reducing nationwide overweightness. The "outlaw food advertising" circus is politicians' feckless ruse.

False Assumption 11: *Enacting food taxation and consumption laws will make people "eat right."* ❧ For decades now we've imposed heavy taxes on cigarettes and liquor. Has it stopped cigarette smoking and liquor drinking? Obviously not. So, why are the proponents of this assumption thinking that taxing "bad" foods will end consumption of "bad" foods when taxing hasn't ended smoking and drinking?

Getting the people of our nation to minimize wrong eating and increase right eating won't happen by outlawing food advertising and piling heavy taxes on "bad" foods. Rather, it will happen when our government leaders enact a national program that equips people with the resources, know-how, and motivation to voluntarily engage in right eating. For more, see Section C (p. **182**).

And, speaking of motivating people to eat right, one of the most powerful motivators would be a leadership *role model* — that is, it would be *every* key person who's working in our federal congressional and executive branches setting an *example* by doing daily right eating and achieving personal healthy-weight living. Such a model would be a big step toward motivating the people of our nation to engage in right eating and healthy-weight living. It would be far more motivating than the "tax bad foods" circus that some politicians are trying to foist on us.

False Assumption 12: *Overweightness is a physical problem, so the solution must be a physical solution.* ❧ For years we've been spending thousands of hours and millions of dollars trying to discover a physical fix to the burgeoning overweightness condition. But we haven't discovered it. Why? Because it doesn't exist. Yes, overweightness is, indeed, a physical issue. But the fix to this physical issue happens to involve a *mind* solution. Enacting this solution is the key to ending overweight living. This book was written to describe the easiest, most enjoyable, most effective form of this solution.

False Assumption 13: *Succeeding at losing weight is the main achievement and most important thing.* ❧ In the world of weight control we have our priorities askew. Losing weight is im-

portant and applaud-worthy but it's not the end of each individual weight story, as most people assume it to be. Rather, it's the *beginning* of the story; it's Chapter 1. What happens next in the years *after* the weight loss is the main thing. This is the big story, the story that needs to be told, and read about, and applauded, because this is when creation of healthy-weight living actually happens. I suggest that if we viewed weight control from this perspective we would be more effective at conquering overweightness and creating both individual and nationwide healthy-weight living.

False Assumption 14: *You don't understand what it takes to create healthy-weight living until you've gained a lot of weight and lost it.* ❧ One of the most entrenched assumptions in the world of weight control is that one doesn't, or perhaps can't, understand what it takes to create healthy-weight living until one has first become hugely overweight and then lost the excess weight. We tend to assume that having this experience somehow endows a person with special insight into the process of healthy weight achievement.

That assumption is false. This is proven by the fact that, at the present time, over ninety percent of people who go through the experience of gaining and then losing a lot of weight eventually become overweight again. So, clearly, if the process of losing a large amount of weight automatically endowed a person with special insight into the process of creating healthy-weight living, everyone who succeeds at losing a large amount of weight would be living out the rest of their life in their healthy-weight range.

So who should we be looking to for a role model? There are two groups of people who have undergone a certain experience that's even more enlightening and noteworthy than that of gaining and then losing a huge amount of weight.

The first group consists of people who decided early in their life that they would live out their life in their healthy-weight range, and then committed their self to doing that, and created a personal life plan or healthy-weight strategy for accomplishing it, and then implemented that strategy throughout their life and achieved lifelong healthy-weight living as a result.

The second group consists of people who began gaining weight at some point in their life and then, after putting on 10 or 20 excess pounds, decided to change the situation and to live out the rest of their life in their healthy-weight range, and then created a personal life plan or healthy-weight living strategy for accomplishing it, and then implemented that strategy for the rest of their life and, as a result, lived out the remainder of their life in their healthy-weight range.

Both these groups fly under the radar, so to speak. We pay little attention to them because, for the most part, the people in these two groups just quietly go about "doing their thing." So no one's noticing their unique accomplishment, and certainly no one's applauding it. And, on the rare occasion when one of these weight winners becomes known, or decides to share their healthy-weight strategy or story, very few people take note of it.

This is too bad, because the people in these two small groups have acquired even more valuable insight into the process of creating healthy-weight living than have those who became highly overweight and lost the weight. These people have discovered — either knowingly or unknowingly, intentionally or non-intentionally — what it takes to achieve lifelong healthy-weight living, and then are *doing it*. They're the ones we should be "studying," listening to, and learning from.

False Assumption 15: *Since 70 percent of us are overweight, 30 percent of us aren't affected by overweightness.* ❧ Federal government survey as of 2017 indicates that about 70 percent of adults (those over age 18) are overweight and 30 percent are non-overweight. These numbers are alarming, yet they likely greatly *under*represent the magnitude of the overweightness situation. Here's why.

The "30% non-overweight" number depicts a slice in time, a moment when a survey occurred. But when we view the overweight situation over a span of years we can see the truth. Which is, many of the people in the "30% non-overweight" category will, in the future, *be overweight.*

The 30% non-overweight category mainly comprises four groups of persons: **(1)** yo-yo dieters who are at the low-weight end of the yo-yo cycle but who will be overweight again in about twelve months, **(2)** young people who are presently non-overweight but will become overweight in just a few years as they live more of "the good life," **(3)** hyper-exercisers who are beating back fat gain with vigorous calorie-burning activity but who will eventually find it doesn't work as they grow older, and **(4)** people who have adopted a lifelong eating management strategy that results in consuming an amount of calories that's equal to the amount their body is metabolizing.

I estimate that groups one through three constitute at least half of the "30% non-overweight" category (which would equal 15% of total population), and group four constitutes the other half (15% of population).

So, to sum up, the magnitude of the overweightness situation isn't accurately portrayed by the tidy "70% overweight, 30% non-overweight" ratio. The reality is, it's likely that about *85 percent* of the population ends up living their life stricken with overweightness (70% + 15% = 85%). So, for about 85 percent of us, becoming overweight isn't a matter of IF — rather, it's a matter of *when* and *how much.*

This is a sobering scenario. So how do we break it? Simply put, we equip, teach, and motivate the people of our nation — and perhaps the world — to do what group 4 is doing. That is, we teach, equip, and motivate them to apply an eating management strategy that enables them to *easily, enjoyably* manage their eating in a way that results in consuming an amount of calories that's equal to the amount their body is metabolizing. A main aim of this book is to explain this process.

False Assumption 16: *Our overweightness is caused by a complex multifactor condition.* ❧ For decades now, governmental bodies, academia, the scientific–medical community, and society-at-large have been seeking the cause of and solution to our growing overweightness. We've sunk thousands of hours and millions of dollars into it. And yet —

by the evidence and by the opinion of some experts — we're no closer today to understanding and discovering the elusive "cause and solution" to our growing weight failure than we were when we started looking for it decades ago.

The only thing that has resulted from it all is a delusion-creating mire of fat-promoting factors (p. **146**), which has led us to the copout conclusion "There's no point in us even trying to personally control our weight."

So, why is it that after all the time and money spent on trying to identify the cause of our over-weightness we haven't found it until now — until the creation of this book? It's because of this. As a nation we've been holding a powerful false assumption: the assumption that weight failure is caused by a *complex multifactor condition*. Holding this assumption has created a bizarre, counterproductive situation. It has made us unable to recognize the real cause of our overweightness. In short, we're not "seeing" this real cause because it's a *simple single-factor* condition instead of being the complex multifactor condition that most researchers assume exists and are looking for.

This simple single-factor condition — explained in False Assumption 1 (p. 146) — happens to be *overperformance of the three-action process of opening one's mouth, inserting food into one's mouth, and swallowing the food.* This is the REAL cause — and also the most productive explanation — of why overweightness exists.

So, why are researchers perpetually not recognizing the real cause of overweightness? The reason is simple. It's because this single-factor explanation contradicts the complex multi-factors assumption held by most weight researchers. Or, put another way, they're not recognizing the obvious simple answer because they're assuming this answer doesn't exist. Or, put still another way, they're not seeing reality because this reality is not what they expect, or want, to see.

All this would be amusing except for one thing. It's sad that we're wasting such vast amounts of time and money in pursuit of trying to discover something that doesn't exist. So, what should we be doing instead? Two things. First, we should cease our feckless pursuit of the imaginary multi-factor fat-causing condition. Second, we should take a portion of the time and money we save by ceasing our pointless pursuit of the non-existent condition and allocate it to doing the only thing that will enable us to achieve both personal and nationwide healthy-weight living. We should equip people with the wherewithal — motivation, resources, and method — for easily guiding themselves each day to right eating and healthy-weight living. For more, see Section C (p. **182**).

Once we escape our false beliefs regarding eating and weight we'll be in position to more quickly achieve nationwide healthy-weight living. The approach of the Weight Success Method ignores and/or circumvents these false beliefs rather than accepting and embracing them. This is one reason why the Method is so effective at creating lifelong healthy-weight living.

CHAPTER 21: Key to Beating the Bad Habit of Unguided Eating

Most people find it hard to end unguided eating. But doing the Weight Success Method makes it easier.

WOULD YOU like to know what's causing most people to engage in unguided eating … and why they find it so hard to free themselves from it? Would you like to know why the Weight Success Method enables one to more easily escape unguided eating and, thereby, more easily create healthy-weight living for life? If so, read on.

The Eating Triggers

Most eating occurs as a habitual response to one of six conditions. I call these conditions *eating triggers*. They are: food, hunger feeling, desire for eating-derived pleasure, time period, situation, and mood. I'll explain.

1 – Food. The presence of food or pictures of food can trigger eating. Also, an aroma of food can do it, too.

2 – Hunger Feeling. The presence of hunger, also known as hunger pang, can trigger eating. It works like this. Hunger is an unpleasant feeling; the desire to remove this unpleasant feeling prompts us to eat.

3 – Desire for Eating-derived Pleasure. A desire to experience pleasure by way of consuming food can trigger eating. When this desire is strong and pertains to a certain type of food we call it a craving. This trigger happens to be a big promoter of unguided eating for many people. The pleasure-priority approach to eating, which is described in Startup Action 6 (p. **39**), derives from the desire to experience eating pleasure.

4 – Time Period. The arrival of a certain time period — such as, for example, lunchtime, dinnertime, snack time — can trigger eating.

5 – Situation. The presence of a certain situation can trigger eating. For examples, a holiday, social event, or tense situation might be an eating trigger for some persons.

6 – Mood: The presence of a certain mood or feeling can trigger eating. For examples, happiness, anxiety, or sadness might be an eating promoter for some persons.

All six triggers don't necessarily apply to every person. Plus, each trigger affects various persons in different ways. For one person a certain trigger might have minimal impact and for another person a huge impact. So, whether a trigger is strong or weak depends on the person.

Three Responses to Eating Triggers

Now we come to the vital point. How a person *responds* to the eating triggers in their life determines whether they live *in* their healthy-weight range or *outside* their healthy-weight range. Most people assume there's only one response to these triggers: automatic, or unguided, eating. But that's not correct. There are *three* possible responses: (1) unguided eating, (2) guided eating, (3) no eating. Here's what's involved with each.

Unguided Eating. In unguided eating we don't guide our eating actions. Instead, the eating triggers do it, especially trigger #1: *the presence of food*. Food items are visual cues. The cues trigger a certain behavior. This certain behavior consists of performing a series of unguided-eating actions that result in consuming the cues. We mostly perform this unguided-eating behavior automatically, or with very little deliberation or conscious direction. (Note: Other names for unguided eating are automatic eating, undirected eating, and non-controlled eating.)

So, unguided eating is a 3-action process. First, we confront food items, which are cues. Second, the food cues trigger an automatic-eating response. Third, we engage in undirected or automatic eating until the cues disappear from being eaten. During this time we aren't thinking about what we're doing. As a result, we're not guiding our eating activity. And, whenever we're not guiding our eating activity, our eating activity is <u>un</u>controlled. Which is why unguided eating leads to overeating and eventual failure at creating lifelong healthy-weight living. So, we should replace unguided eating with guided eating.

Guided Eating. In guided eating *we* guide the eating process. Meaning, instead of the food items determining what and how much we eat, *we* do it. This might sound hard to do, but it's not. You can easily create guided eating any time you want. All you need do is apply a certain 3-action process, which we call *Guided Eating Process.* (Other names for guided eating are directed eating and controlled eating.) This Process is described in Daily Action 5 (p. **56**). Guided eating is a major key to replacing overweight living with healthy-weight living for life.

> **Note:** In this book the word "eating" encompasses drinking. And the word "food" encompasses beverages. So wherever you read the terms "eating" and "food" know that it includes drinking and beverages.

No Eating. In addition to unguided eating and guided eating there's a third possible response to the eating triggers: no eating.

Each response produces a certain outcome. *Unguided eating,* done daily or frequently, leads to living <u>above</u> your healthy-weight range. *Guided eating,* done daily or frequently, leads to living <u>in</u> your healthy-weight range. And, *no eating,* done in moderation, might also lead to living *in* your healthy-weight range, <u>or</u> when done to excess lead to living *below* your healthy-weight range.

The Habit of Unguided Eating

A person's response to any particular eating trigger is determined one of two ways: either by deliberate choice or by habit. A *habit* is an automatic frequently-repeated behavior or activity. So, the *habit of unguided eating* is unguided eating done automatically and repeatedly.

Most people respond to the eating triggers of their life not by deliberate choice but by habit. Further, the particular habit that's most in play is the habit of unguided eating. Which means, for

most people, every time an eating trigger appears they automatically engage in habit-driven unguided eating. Unfortunately, this ultimately results in overweight living. So, a main Cause–Effect Dynamic of Overweight Living is this:

Eating Triggers prompt **Habit-driven Unguided Eating** which causes Overweight Living

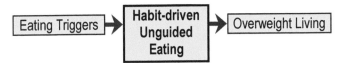

This means, to more easily live the rest of your life in your healthy-weight range you need to override or nullify the habit of unguided eating. And, then, replace that habit with deliberate guided eating and, eventually, a guided-eating habit. By doing this the unguided-eating problem would be instantly solved.

But this is easier said than done. Why so? Because most likely your habit of unguided eating is a *strong* habit. And why is it strong? Because the more a habit is repeated the stronger it becomes. So, if you're like most folks, by the time you decide to switch from unguided eating to guided eating your habit of unguided eating has been repeated for *numerous* years, which comprises *thousands* of days and <u>tens</u> *of thousands* of unguided eating sessions. The result of all this repetition is: Your habit of unguided eating has become a strong, *deeply engrained* habit. Which means, for many people the strength of their unguided-eating habit is a main impediment to easily conquering overweightness and creating healthy-weight living.

A Habit Is a Beast of Two Components

In addition to the habit of unguided eating being strong, most people don't know how to defeat an unwanted habit. This is because they don't know the anatomy of a habit. They don't realize that every habit consists of two parts: a physical component and a mental component. The physical component, which I call *action-habit,* is a certain automatic repeating physical activity. The mental component, which I call *mind-habit,* is a certain automatic repeating mental process. Now here's the big point:

The mind-habit underlies and drives the action-habit. It works like this.

Two-part Anatomy of a Habit

Action-habit Component
Automatic repeating physical activity

- - - - - ⬆ - - - - -

Mind-habit Component
Automatic repeating mental process
that underlies and drives the action-habit

So, to shut down an action-habit, or automatic repeating physical activity, you must shut down the mind-habit, or automatic repeating mental process that's driving the physical activity. Which means, to shut down habit-driven unguided eating you must shut down, or override, the mental process that's causing it.

So for most folks the situation is this. The combination of the unguided-eating habit's strength plus lack of understanding of how habits work makes it a major struggle to override the habit of unguided eating for most persons. This, in turn, causes them to eventually give up the battle.

The Solution

So, how does one solve this problem? You involve your *whole* mind, or both conscious <u>and</u> subconscious mind, in your daily pursuit of living in your healthy-weight range. When you do this it brings the faculties of your subconscious mind into your pursuit of healthy-weight living. This results in shutting down, or at least mitigating, the mind-habit component of unguided eating. Which, in turn, results in shutting down or mitigating the action-habit component, or the automatic unguided-eating response to the eating triggers of your life. Finally, as previously stated, the easiest way to involve your whole mind in your weight success pursuit is do the Weight Success Method.

Summation

To conclude this chapter I provide a summary in the form of three infographics, starting with this one.

How Overweight Living Comes About

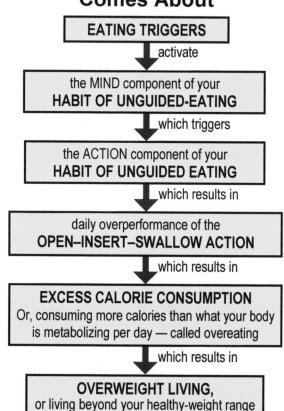

Most people don't realize it, but the process depicted in this infographic is what makes weight gain happen so easily. It's also what makes weight loss seem so hard. And, lastly, it's what makes weight maintenance, or living in one's healthy-weight range, seem even harder.

But there's a way to break free of this dynamic. It involves something you're already familiar with: the Weight Success Method. Here's the infographic for it, titled "Easiest Way to Beat the Habit of Unguided Eating."

Easiest Way to Beat the Habit of Unguided Eating

Each day do the five daily actions of the
WEIGHT SUCCESS METHOD

which produces

increased RIGHT-EATING **FOCUS** by the *conscious* mind
<u>and</u> increased RIGHT-EATING **COMMUNICATION**
delivered to the *subconscious* mind

which creates

WHOLE MIND INVOLVEMENT or having both conscious
<u>and</u> subconscious mind involved in healthy-weight living

which results in

your mind creating thoughts and feelings that guide you to
GUIDED EATING (in place of habit-driven unguided eating)

which results in

CORRECT CALORIE CONSUMPTION
Or, eating right foods in right amounts — called Right Eating

which results in

you living most or all of the rest of your days in your
healthy-weight range – called **HEALTHY-WEIGHT LIVING**

> For an in-depth explanation of how FOCUS and SELF-COMMUNICATION create whole mind involvement, go to the *Why the Weight Success Method Gets Your Whole Mind Involved* chapter (p. **129**).

Here's a concluding way to view this. Your habit of unguided eating is on a mission to make you overeat. And, as long as you're not doing anything to thwart this mission it will succeed at its mission. Which means, either *you* direct your eating <u>or</u> the *habit of unguided eating* will direct it. And, when the habit of unguided eating is directing it you *will* end up overeating.

In case you might be interested in it, here's the above infographic in a summary sentence: Doing the Weight Success Method each day produces daily Right-eating Focus and Right-eating Communication which, in turn, creates daily Whole Mind Involvement in pursuit of healthy-weight living, which results in daily Right Eating that ultimately results in correct calorie consumption and lifelong Healthy-weight Living.

The Habit vs. You

Here's another way to view it. You and your *Habit of Unguided Eating* are rival contestants in a daily wrestling match. Each day the Habit shows up for a showdown between it and you. Depending on your resolve, it might be a short match, like, say, 20 seconds, or it might last an entire day. But either way, before day's end one of you will come out on top, dominating the other. When the Habit of Unguided Eating comes out on top, you end up engaging in overeating for the day. When YOU come out on top, you end up doing guided eating, which results in <u>non</u>-overeating for the day.

Now here's the key point. You have a secret weapon that makes the difference: your mind. When you go into the match using only the "conscious half" of your mind you usually lose. But when you involve your whole mind — or both conscious <u>and</u> subconscious mind — you win. This almost always makes it a short contest, with you coming out on top. So each day *you* determine how it will be, and whether the winner will be **IT** (your Habit of Unguided Eating) or **YOU.** Here's the infographic for it (next page).

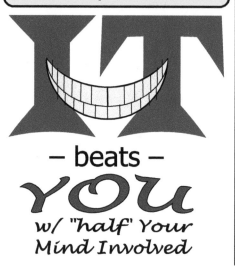

IT beats *YOU* when you use "half" your mind.

– beats –
YOU
w/ "half" Your Mind Involved

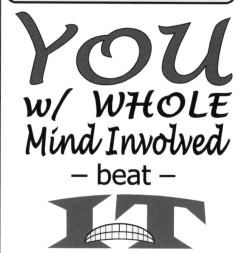

YOU beat **IT** when you use your WHOLE mind.

YOU
w/ WHOLE Mind Involved
– beat –
IT

AND, doing Weight Success Actions — such as the five daily actions of the Weight Success Method — every day *greatly assists* you with involving your whole mind — or both conscious <u>and</u> subconscious mind — every day.

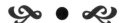

For decades now we've been spending thousands of hours and millions of dollars each year searching for the solution to individual and global overweightness. But prior to this book we haven't found it. We haven't found it because we've been assuming it involves anything but what it actually involves, which is each person's **MIND** and the capability of that mind to **SUCCEED** at creating ongoing weight success.

CHAPTER 22: How the Weight Success Method Enhances Your Life Journey

This is how the Weight Success Method makes your weight success journey feel easier and more natural, and also more fulfilling.

THE 19 SUCCESS DRIVERS described in Chapter 2 (p. **23**) are outstandingly effective at creating achievement of lifelong healthy-weight living. But upon completing one of the precursor manuscripts for this book I got a suspicion that maybe there was even more going on than that. This prompted some Internet research. I had heard of a relatively new field of psychology called *positive psychology,* but knew nothing about it. So I typed "positive psychology" into my Google search bar and went on a voyage of discovery.

After clicking through a few sites I ended up at one titled authentichappiness.org. This appeared to be the epicenter of the positive psychology movement. I discovered that a founding pioneer in the field is a professor Martin Seligman of University of Pennsylvania — a.k.a. Penn.

At this site I viewed some videos, read some articles, and filled out a couple questionnaires, or tests. I also discovered that Seligman had recently published a book titled *Flourish: A Visionary New Understanding of Happiness and Well-being.* I decided that this is what I needed to be reading. So I ordered a copy from Amazon. I also ordered another book that had been mentioned on the website — a book titled *Flow: The Psychology of Optimal Experience* by a professor Mihaly Csikszentmihalyi of Claremont Graduate University. (Note: Csikszentmihalyi is pronounced CHEEK-sent-me-hi.) And, I ordered a third book — titled *A Primer in Positive Psychology* — by a professor Christopher Peterson of University of Michigan.

In a few days the books arrived. First I read *Flourish,* then *Flow,* then *A Primer in Positive Psychology.* I found each to be interesting and enlightening.

After just a few pages into *Flourish* I came upon a seminal concept. That being, a main tenet of positive psychology is that a person experiences well-being by having five main elements in their life: Positive emotion, Engagement, Relationships (of the positive kind), Meaning, and Accomplishment. The acronym for these five things is PERMA. And the main idea is: The more PERMA — or Positive emotion, Engagement, Relationships, Meaning, and Accomplishment — a person has in their life, the more well-being the person experiences.

I then examined the Weight Success Method in light of the PERMA model. To my astonishment, the Weight Success Method correlated closely with the PERMA model. I discovered that doing the Method results in *expanded actualization* of four of the five elements of the model and, with a little innovation, even all five.

Then a stunning realization hit me. Perhaps this is a reason why creating healthy-weight living with the Weight Success Method seems so easy and natural. It's because gaining healthy-weight living via the Method not only results in creating a "new" physical body it also results in creating expanded psychological well-being, or fulfillment, in a person's life. Or, put another way, it makes one's weight management journey to be an enhancer of the life journey. Which means, it turns weight management from a "life detracting activity" — which is how most view it — into a "life enhancing activity."

Then another realization struck me. Those few people who are seemingly doing right eating easily, enjoyably, and automatically might be doing right eating in a way that results in expanding one or more of the PERMA elements in their life. Conversely, those who are finding right eating to be painful and hard to do might be doing it in a way that results in no expansion, or perhaps even diminishment, of the PERMA elements in their life.

So, I'll now describe each of the five PERMA elements, and explain how doing the Weight Success Method results in expansion of that element. Also, in some cases I'll describe some additional actions a person could take to expand a certain element even further.

Note: In examining the five elements I'm doing it in a slightly different order than the PERMA model. The order I'm using is P-A-R-M-E. I'm doing so because "E" is where I want to end up in the discussion.

Positive Emotion

The first element of the PERMA model is positive emotion. Upon reviewing some literature on the model I soon realized that none of the sources defined the term "positive emotion." What's more, a few didn't even give examples. But some did. Here's a combined list of examples of positive emotions cited in positive psychology literature: pleasure, happiness, joy, satisfaction, gratitude, hope, serenity, kindness, contentment, comfort, interest, pride, excitement, amusement, inspiration, awe, ecstasy, and love.

So, to promote clarity of discussion I now provide this formal definition.

Positive emotion is any harm-free emotion or feeling that one enjoys having.

NOTE: Harm-free = Doesn't derive from doing harm to oneself or others, and doesn't result in harm to oneself or others

So now you likely want to know how the Weight Success Method expands the amount of positive emotion, or enjoyment, in a person's life. Well, you may have already discovered it. The *Why the Weight Success Method Is Enjoyable* chapter (p. **123**) explains it in detail. It's a full description, based on my personal experiences, of the enjoyment that can be derived from doing the Weight Success Method.

Now here's an important thing to know. Positive emotion, or enjoyment and gratification, that's

derived from the Weight Success Method comes two ways: (1) from realizing the desired *outcome*, or from living in one's healthy-weight range and deriving weight success benefits from it, and (2) from the *process* of creating the outcome. What distinguishes the Weight Success Method from most other weight management programs is Way #2: deriving enjoyment from *the process*.

To illustrate, here's a summation of the enjoyment and gratification I personally derive from doing the Weight Success Method. Some items come from the outcome and some from the process. (Again, for a full discussion go to the Why the Weight Success Method Is Enjoyable chapter, page **123**.)

Enjoyment Derived from the Weight Success Method

Stated in summary, doing the Weight Success Method expands the amount of enjoyment, or positive emotions, in my life because doing the Method results in the following enjoyment-creating experiences: (a) achieving and seeing daily personal progress, (b) delivering and receiving positive self-reinforcement, (c) triumphing over occasional adversity or setbacks, (d) being director of my eating, (e) daily focusing on an exciting ultimate goal, and (f) feeling like a winner by performing daily winning actions.

I also derive enjoyment and satisfaction from (g) succeeding at living in my healthy-weight range, which makes me feel like a high-achiever, (h) realizing exciting weight success benefits from living at my healthy weight, and (i) maintaining awareness of those benefits on a daily basis.

And, finally, I derive enjoyment and gratification from (j) the act of improving my self and my life by pursuing a productive activity in place of a counterproductive one, or by living in my healthy-weight range rather than outside it, and from (k) being a living example that achieving easier healthy-weight living is *doable*, thereby inspiring others to "give it a go."

Items (a) through (f) occur from the *process*, or from performing the actions involved in doing the

Weight Success Method. Items (g) through (k) come from the *outcome,* or from having accomplished the desired results connected to the Method.

In short, by doing the Weight Success Method you can *expand* your amount of enjoyment and satisfaction, or the positive emotion element, in your life. This can occur in various ways throughout each day and over your lifetime.

Accomplishment

A look at some positive psychology literature — in particular, Seligman's book *Flourish* (pgs. 18–20) — reveals a clear description of what's involved with the accomplishment element. Deriving from that information I put forth the following definition.

> *Accomplishment is the progressive realization of success, winning, achievement, or mastery in a particular chosen activity or endeavor.*

The literature describes several characteristics pertaining to accomplishment, as follows.

Accomplishment can be for its own sake. That is, for no other purpose than to achieve success, mastery, or a winning position in a particular activity or endeavor. But, in certain cases accomplishment can contribute to expansion of other PERMA elements, such as positive emotion, meaning, or relationships.

Further, it can occur both on-the-job and off-the-job, or at work, home, and in recreational pursuits.

Still further, it can be performed individually or as part of a group.

To create accomplishment with a particular endeavor it helps to apply as many of the 19 Success Drivers as possible. You already know about these drivers; they're described in Chapter 2 (p. **23**.)

Accomplishment Derived from the Weight Success Method

So how, exactly, does doing the Weight Success Method expand the amount of accomplishment in a person's life? It does it by enabling the person to have these four experiences:

1. Each day, or most days, getting a desired weight reading at the daily weigh-in (Daily Action 1– Weighing);

2. Whenever an <u>un</u>desired weight reading happens, triumphing over adversity, or converting the setback into a progress action (Daily Action 2B–Correction);

3. Acquiring the weight success benefits attached to creating healthy-weight living, and also maintaining a daily awareness of those benefits; and

4. Creating lifelong healthy-weight living, a notable accomplishment, indeed — a feat that proves *mastery* of a special life pursuit and imparts the status of "lifelong healthy-weight *winner.*"

Those are four ways the Weight Success Method can expand the amount of accomplishment in a person's life.

How to Expand Accomplishment Even Further

But, even with all that, it's possible to further expand the accomplishment element in your weight success journey. Here are four ways.

1. *ENHANCE the Weight Success Method.* You can do this by customizing certain parts of the five daily actions. In describing the five daily actions I noted where you might tweak, or customize, an action if you so chose. For example, in doing Daily Action 2A–Reinforcement you might expand on the wording of the Thank You, Keep It Up message. And, in doing Daily Action 3–Benefits Directive you might include various enhancements to the Weight Success Benefits Directive and also apply changes in delivery style (see the "Enhancing the Directive" section and the "Apply Creative Delivery Techniques" section in the Detailed Instructions for the

Weight Success Benefits Directive chapter, page **85**). And, in doing Daily Action 4–Goal Statement you might experiment with delivering the Healthy-weight Goal Statement in different ways. Finally, in Daily Action 5–Guided Eating you might use enhanced wording for your guided-eating self-talk. Depending on how you approach it, these enhancement actions can further expand the feeling of accomplishment to be derived from doing the Weight Success Method.

2. *ADD TO the Weight Success Method.* You can do this by including *optional additional* mind motivation actions along with doing the five daily actions. The *Six More Mind Motivators* chapter (p. **110**) provides six optional additional mind motivators. You can include any one you like. And, you can modify, improvise, or enhance any of them, if you like.

3. *DO the optional Weight Success Actions Scorecard.* This can be a great way to expand the feeling of accomplishment in your weight success journey. If you're one who likes "scoring points," recording what you accomplish, and breaking personal-best records, this is for you. It's in Chapter 27 (p. **174**). Also, doing the Win-Day Calendar, contained in Chapter 27, is an additional way to expand the feeling of accomplishment. And, finally, if you are presently in weight-reduction mode, doing the Weight-reduction Success Graph can bring a feeling of accomplishment, as well (in Ch. 27).

4. *BE CREATIVE in selecting or creating your preferred dietary program.* As you know by now, you have a choice of what dietary program you apply to your weight success journey. It can be one of the established bona fide programs on the market or it can be a program of your own design — your choice. For some people, applying their own custom-designed dietary program might enhance the feeling of accomplishment derived from their weight success journey. For others, going with one of the established bona fide programs is the best, or most productive, way to go. You're the one who determines which is best for you.

In short, by pursuing creation of healthy-weight living via a full, whole-hearted application of the Weight Success Method — plus perhaps taking advantage of the many ways to enhance and add to the Method — you can greatly *expand* the accomplishment element in your life.

Relationships

As with the positive emotions element, I failed to find a tidy definition of the term "positive relationships." So I provide this formal definition.

*A **positive relationship** is a harm-free regularly-occurring interaction between two or more persons, with the interaction mainly involving constructive activity such as mutually enjoyable conversation, meaningful two-way dialogue, inspiring or positively reinforcing words and actions, and the act of treating each other in a thoughtful manner, or in a way you would like to be treated if you were in their place.*

NOTE: Harm-free = Doesn't result in harm to oneself or others

Of the five PERMA elements, creating positive relationships is the one least impacted by doing the Weight Success Method. This is because the Method has been designed to be a do-it-yourself activity. I made it this way because I don't want your success and my success in the pursuit of healthy-weight living to be dependent on having a certain relationship with others.

But, if you so chose, you could do things that would make performance of the Weight Success Method promote expansion of positive relationships.

Creating Positive Relationships While Doing the Weight Success Method

There are at least two ways a person might expand the relationships element in their life via doing the Weight Success Method.

1. For your preferred dietary program, adopt one of the established dietary programs that includes positive interaction with coaches and co-dieters.

2. Create a "healthy-weight achievement group" consisting of you and one or more others who are pursuing the Weight Success Method, or otherwise pursuing the goal of living in their healthy-weight range.

For either option to qualify as a positive relationship it likely would need to meet the above formal definition of a positive relationship. Meaning, it should include relationship-building activities such as constructive communication, inspiring words or positive reinforcement, sharing of progress actions, ideas, and discoveries, and perhaps even some group exercise activity.

In short, by forming a positive relationship with one or more persons, with one of the goals of the relationship being creation of healthy-weight living, you would *expand* the positive relationships element in your life, and also likely make creating healthy-weight living even easier and more enjoyable.

Meaning

Okay, sounds simple, but what exactly *is* meaning? Like the prior three PERMA elements, a tidy definition is hard to find. In his book *Flow,* Csikszentmihalyi devotes the entire last chapter, titled "The Making of Meaning," to explaining it in detail and depth. In the third paragraph of the chapter it says this:

> "If a person sets out to achieve a difficult enough goal, from which all other goals logically follow, and if he or she invests all energy in developing skills to reach that goal, then actions and feelings will be in harmony, and the separate parts of life will fit together — and each activity will 'make sense' in the present, as well as in view of the past and of the future. In such a way, it is possible to give meaning to one's entire life."

For a shorter definition I turn to Seligman. In his book *Flourish* he defines meaning (by way of a parenthetical phrase) as "belonging to and serving something that you believe is bigger than self."

So that's the long and short of it. For this discussion I split the difference, and do a little paraphrasing and creative adaptation, to derive this formal definition.

> ***Meaning*** *is the situation of perceiving one's life as existing for fulfillment of a certain worthwhile overriding purpose, or ultimate goal, with that goal being associated with serving or enhancing something bigger than one's self.*

So how can a person use the pursuit of healthy-weight living to enhance meaning in their life? Or, put another way, how can they use the pursuit of healthy-weight living to enhance their perspective or belief that their life exists for fulfillment of a certain worthwhile overriding purpose?

Enhancing Life Meaning via Your Pursuit of Healthy-weight Living

From my perspective, the key to making the pursuit of healthy-weight living — or any personal development activity — contribute to enhancement of life meaning is to adopt a life perspective that embraces personal development as an activity that enhances or serves a higher purpose, or "something bigger than oneself."

The easiest, most effective way to explain how one might do this is by citing an example. And the example I know best is me. So here's the approach I personally use for creating overall life meaning and, in particular, for making my pursuit of healthy-weight living contribute to enhancing that meaning. It involves adoption of the following seven assumptions.

1. I assume there's a God. I realize that in the eyes of some this assumption might appear old-fashioned or wrong-headed, but I've found it to be the simplest, most effective starting point for creating and enhancing meaning in my life.

2. I assume that God is a universal spiritual being on an endless journey of conceptualization and actualization, which I call *creation journey* for short. I assume that a result of this creation journey is the evolving universe and everything in it.

3. I assume that part of this creation journey is the creation of life and the evolvement of life forms. I further assume that on planet Earth the present apex of this evolvement of life forms is human beings.

4. I assume that God made this evolution of human beings to happen for a certain purpose: specifically, to create beings that can appreciate, contribute to, and be part of his creation journey.

5. I assume that to enable humans to contribute to this journey God made the human species to possess a mini version, or micro extension, of some of God's powers. For reference purpose I call these powers *spiritual powers,* although they could be called spiritual faculties, instead. From my viewpoint, these spiritual powers include (a) the power to deliberately focus, (b) the power to discern, (c) the power to choose, in particular the power to choose what to think, to feel, and to do, (d) the power to depict and describe, (e) the power to create, hold, and act on a belief, including the power to act as-if, (f) the power to appreciate and to express thanks, (g) the power to look toward the future and survey possible outcomes and alternatives, and (h) the power to conceptualize and actualize — a.k.a. the power to achieve and create success — that is, the power to create an <u>actual</u> situation that corresponds to a certain <u>imagined desired</u> situation, or goal.

6. I assume that there are three main ways that each human can contribute to God's creation journey: (1) by performing acts that contribute to them becoming a finer person, (2) by performing acts that contribute to them creating a more beneficial life, and (3) by helping others do the same. I call these three actions God-enhancement Actions 1, 2, and 3.

7. Finally, I assume that the realization of healthy-weight living — or living most or all of our days in our healthy-weight range — is an activity that promotes *all three* of these God-enhancement actions.

In short, adopting the above seven assumptions is how I impart greater meaning to my life. And, it's also how I enhance the meaning of my weight success journey, which, in turn, further expands the meaning element in my life.

Engagement (or Flow)

Upon first encounter, I found engagement — a.k.a. flow — to be the only one of the five PERMA elements that was confusing. The confusion derived from disparate descriptions of what it is. Here, for example, are seven descriptions, reproduced verbatim, from six pieces of literature.

1. *Engagement = being fully absorbed in activities that use your skills and challenge you.*

2. *Engagement refers to involvement in activities that draw and build upon one's interests. Csikszentmihalyi explains true engagement as flow, a feeling of intensity that leads to a sense of ecstasy and clarity.*

3. *Engagement refers to a deep psychological connection (e.g., being interested, engaged, and absorbed) to a particular activity, organization, or cause.*

4. *Engagement is about being totally absorbed (in a flow) by a present task where time and self-consciousness cease to exist.*

5. *Engagement – being completely absorbed in activities.*

6. *Flow: the psychological state that accompanies highly engaging activities.*

7. *Flow can be described as the experience of working at full capacity.*

Taken in total, this list of descriptions is befuddling. It also seems to indicate that, as a group, positive psychology practitioners seem to lack a unified concept of what engagement is or entails.

So, in an attempt to clarify things I returned to the book *Flow.* Now let me take a second to tell you about this book. If you like easy-reading fluff this book's not your type. It's a densely packed tome. But the good news is: It's a gold mine of intriguing research, insights, observations, and prescriptions. I typically read non-fiction books with pencil in hand so I can mark the occasional good thought or key point. With *Flow*, I found myself seemingly marking entire pages and sections.

So I re-opened *Flow* and leafed through it looking for a tidy definition of flow — a.k.a. engagement. And, guess what, I couldn't find one (which doesn't necessarily mean it's not there but, rather, it could be my old eyes didn't spot it).

So I reconciled myself to constructing a definition based on the information in the book. In Part B, in a section titled "The Elements of Enjoyment," the book describes eight components the author calls "the phenomenology of enjoyment." I then paraphrased and condensed it. What resulted is the following description.

When people reflect on how it feels when their experience is most positive, they mention at least one, and often all, of the following:

1. it's an activity that's <u>challenging but doable</u>;

2. they're able to <u>focus totally</u> on the activity, to the point that doing it becomes spontaneous or automatic;

3. the activity has <u>clear goals</u>;

4. they get <u>immediate feedback</u> on how they're doing;

5. they pursue the activity with a <u>deep, effortless involvement</u> (that excludes everyday worries and concerns);

6. they can <u>exercise control</u> over their actions;

7. they're <u>free of self-consciousness</u> — that is, thoughts about their self disappear; and

8. they're so involved they <u>lose track of time</u>.

After viewing this paraphrase a realization hit me. When distilled to its essence, what this describes is a situation in which a person has their *whole mind involved* in the performance of a certain activity, or in pursuit of a certain goal. By "whole mind involved" I mean: all the faculties of their mind that contribute to creating optimal performance in that particular activity. This includes both conscious <u>and</u> subconscious mind faculties.

So how does this relate to the prior list of eight factors that constitute the phenomenology of enjoyment? Like this. Items 1, 2, 3, 4, and 6 describe characteristics that foster, or enable, a person to have their whole mind involved in the performance of an activity. Items 5, 7, and 8 describe what a person experiences as a result of having their whole mind involved.

So, from my perspective the situation of engagement, or flow, happens whenever a person has all the performance-enhancing faculties of their whole mind — that is, both conscious and subconscious mind — involved in a certain activity or in pursuit of a certain goal. As such, this leads me to the following definition.

> ***Engagement*** *— a.k.a. flow — is the situation of having all the performance-enhancing faculties of one's whole mind involved in optimal performance of a certain activity or in optimal pursuit of a certain goal.*
>
> | NOTE: "all the performance-enhancing faculties of one's whole mind" = all the faculties of one's mind, both conscious and subconscious, that contribute to creating optimal performance of a certain activity or optimal pursuit of a certain goal

So, referring back to the eight elements of "phenomenology of enjoyment," described in the book *Flow*, we could say: For an activity to be optimally conducive to engagement, or optimally conducive to whole mind involvement, that activity should possess the following eight characteristics: (1) be a challenging but doable activity, (2) enable a person to focus totally on its performance, (3) involve clear goals, (4) provide immediate feedback, (5) enable deep, effortless involvement (that excludes everyday worries and concerns), (6) enable self-direction, or the opportunity to exercise control over one's actions, (7) enable non-self-conscious involvement, or doing the activity free of self-consciousness, and (8) allow for uninterrupted performance, or performance that proceeds without interruption by time or any other focus-distracting factor.

Further, Csikszentmihalyi, Seligman, and Peterson, in their respective books *Flow* and

Flourish and *A Primer in Positive Psychology*, describe a further condition for promoting engagement. They point out that maximal engagement occurs when a person's maximal talents or skills exactly match the challenges presented by the activity.

And why is this match between maximal skills and challenges necessary? Because, when a person's challenge-solving skills greatly exceed the challenges encountered, boredom results. And, when challenge-solving skills are inadequate for resolving the challenges encountered, frustration results. And, when either of these two conditions exists, a person can't get their whole mind involved in performing the activity.

Now here's a key point. Many persons quit the pursuit of weight control due to frustration, or due to a lack of skills that enable them to resolve the challenges they encounter. But the Weight Success Method equips a person with the tools to overcome the challenges involved in this pursuit, thereby removing the frustration and enabling engagement to happen.

> NOTE: As you've seen, the words "engagement" and "flow" are synonyms. Some writers use "engagement," others use "flow." For simplicity, from here on I'm going to use the word **"engagement."** But you should keep in mind that what I'm talking about is what some call "flow."

Engagement and Weight Success Journey

In most cases, when discussing the concept of engagement the writer describes it in the context of a discrete activity — that is, in relation to an activity that has a beginning point and ending point, or involves a distinct period of time that occurs within a certain day. The period of time might be just a few minutes, in which case it's called microflow. Or, it might go for a few hours.

But, sometimes a writer implies that the concept also applies to an ongoing activity, or to a pursuit that extends over months, or years, or even a lifetime.

For example, in *Flow* Csikszentmihalyi starts by mainly discussing the engagement experience as a discrete activity, such as might occur in activities

like rock climbing, chess match, performing a sport, playing music, doing artistic painting, and so forth. But as the book progresses the discussion gradually morphs into focusing more on engagement in *ongoing* activities and eventually ends up discussing engagement in the life journey.

So, this raises a question: Is engagement in an ongoing activity the same as engagement in a discrete activity? My answer would be: Yes and No. In certain basic ways they're alike. Both involve a clear goal, frequent feedback, focus on the task, control over actions, and maximal utilization of certain skills for resolving challenges and gaining goal achievement. In short, both require a type of whole mind involvement.

But in some peripheral ways they differ. For example, in describing discrete-activity engagement some writers cite the characteristic of time distortion — such as, for example, thinking that only a few minutes have elapsed when actually, say, an hour has gone by. Another thing cited as a characteristic of discrete-activity engagement is loss of self-consciousness. Still another is "merging of action and awareness." None of these things exist as characteristics of ongoing-activity engagement, or at least not to the same extent as with discrete-activity engagement.

With the similarities and differences between discrete-activity engagement and ongoing-activity engagement in mind, I propose that a concept of ongoing-activity engagement can be applied to the pursuit of healthy-weight living. And, I further believe, when one pursues healthy-weight living in a state of ongoing-activity engagement that something good happens: creating healthy-weight living becomes easier and more enjoyable.

So, what are the factors that create, or promote, engagement in the performance of an ongoing activity? You've likely already encountered them. They're the 19 Success Drivers listed in the Success Drivers section (p. **23**). When a person applies these nineteen factors to an important ongoing activity that extends over years or a lifetime, that person becomes engaged with the activity in a way that's absorbing, attention-focusing, performance-enhancing, and gratifying — a situation that I call *ongoing-activity engagement*.

Again, the result of this type of engagement is that performance of the activity and achievement of the desired outcome become easier and more automatic. So, what's the easiest way to involve the 19 success drivers in your pursuit of healthy-weight living? You already know: It's do the Weight Success Method. When you fully apply the Weight Success Method to the pursuit of healthy-weight living, you end up pursuing healthy-weight living with whole mind involvement, or ongoing-activity engagement. Or, put yet another way, you get your conscious mind and subconscious mind synced up and working together in pursuit of achieving the goal of you living the rest of your life in your healthy-weight range.

Summing Up

Briefly put, here's how doing the Weight Success Method expands your amount of well-being. It's based on the PERMA model.

First, when you pursue healthy-weight living with the Weight Success Method you end up expanding the amount of enjoyment, or *Positive Emotion,* in your life. Second, you expand the amount of ongoing-activity *Engagement* in your life. Third, if you apply the Weight Success Method in conjunction with other people you would likely expand the amount of positive *Relationships* in your life. Fourth, if you hold a certain "life meaning paradigm" that embraces personal improvement as a noble activity, then pursuing healthy-weight living via the Weight Success Method contributes to expanding *Meaning* in your life. And, fifth, creating healthy-weight living via doing the Weight Success Method expands the amount of *Accomplishment* in your life.

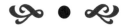

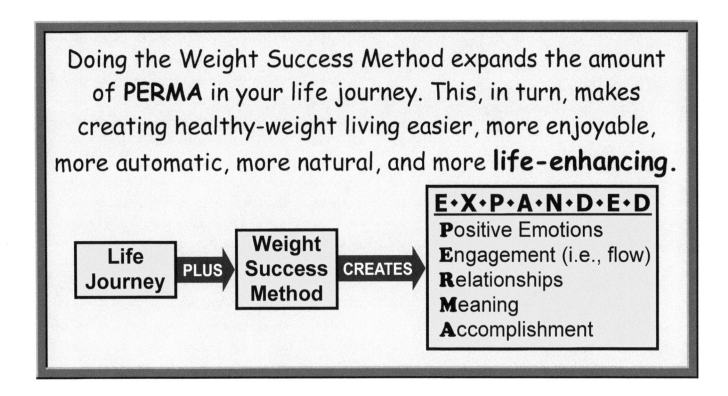

CHAPTER 23: The No-change Secret of Maintenance Achievement

Here's a little-known type of achievement that enables lifelong healthy weight living and also maximal life journey success.

WHERE I LIVE there's a certain ice cream parlor that's especially popular and successful. It has great product, super service, charming décor, and conscientious staff.

I was there one day enjoying a vanilla malt (they have the best in town) when suddenly the owner came out to clear a couple tables. Often when I have a chance to speak to a business owner I pose a certain question. So I said, "You have an excellent business here. Tell me, if you would, what's the secret to your success?"

There were a couple seconds of silence. Then he gave me an answer I'd never heard before and haven't heard since. He said, "No change."

I must have looked puzzled, so he elaborated. "We have a winning formula here. It has been working year after year since the 1960s. My parents started it and I inherited it. MY JOB is to make sure *nothing changes* ... to make sure we keep doing what we've been doing and to preserve the business the way it is today. Staying the same, or not changing, is the secret to our success."

What makes this perspective unique is that very few businesses — indeed, very few people — have as their goal "staying the same." Instead, whenever the subject of success or achievement comes up it's always defined in terms of *change*. That is, it's described in terms of changing one's self or situation from a present state to some other state. Both individually and societally, we have become "wired" to view success and achievement in terms of how much change we make in going from a present situation to a new situation. Change, or moving from situation A to situation B, is what we think of when we hear the word "achievement." I call this *change achievement.*

But there's another form of achievement, which most folks have no experience with. It's what the ice cream parlor owner described. It's the achievement of staying the same, or continuing to do what one is presently doing. I call this *maintenance achievement.* It's the opposite of change achievement. With change achievement, success derives from creating certain change; but with maintenance achievement, success derives from creating <u>no</u> change.

Change achievement is imbedded in our culture. We have books, courses, and methodologies that tell us how to create it. So most everyone has at least an inkling of how to create it. But, maintenance achievement is a mystery. Virtually no one knows how to create it. And herein lies a paradox that's driving ultimate weight failure. In weight maintenance mode, the way we succeed is by creating *no-change,* or staying the same. Oddly, most folks think this can be achieved by "non-action" or "doing nothing." But that's incorrect. Staying the same, or creating no-change, requires as much deliberate focus and action as creating the condition of change. I call this the *no-change secret.* Most folks are unaware of it, which is a major reason why most persons are ineffective at creating the no-change situation required for achieving lifelong weight maintenance, otherwise known as "making weight loss stick."

This situation has been causing us to conclude that weight maintenance is tougher than weight reduction. But this is incorrect. Actually, doing weight maintenance is *easier* than doing weight reduction <u>if</u> you know how to succeed at creating weight maintenance. But most folks don't. So we've been achieving a modicum of success at losing weight and failing miserably at keeping it off.

How do we solve this problem? Do the Weight Success Method. It's specially designed to cause you to take the actions that result in you accomplishing *no*-change after you've succeeded at losing weight and entering your healthy-weight range. Or, put another way, it's specially designed for enacting *both* change achievement involved in creating weight loss <u>and</u> maintenance achievement involved in creating lifelong healthy-weight living. As such, it's <u>the</u> tool by which you can more easily get into your desired weight range *and then easily stay there* the rest of your life.

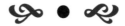

> As a people, we applaud persons for the amount of weight they lose. That's fine. But while doing that, we should be giving standing ovations for the number of years a person keeps that weight off. Losing weight is commendable. But **maintaining** one's healthy weight is a truly exceptional accomplishment. So, allow yourself to have a good feeling from living in your healthy-weight range **every** day you do it.

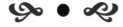

Just Keep Doing Essential

Weight Success Actions

Every Day ... and Lifelong Weight Success will be Yours.

CHAPTER 24: Expanded Weight Success Benefits

Living in your healthy-weight range produces many benefits, which have been previously described. But, amazingly, there are even more benefits to be gained from your weight success journey.

A MAIN RESULT of weight management is a "new" body — specifically, a body that weighs in your desired weight range. This new body and the benefits that come with it are the main outcome of your weight success pursuit.

But, as important as these benefits are, they're not the only possible good outcome to be gained from your weight success journey. There are at least eight possible extra benefits. You might derive one or more — or perhaps all.

1st Possible Benefit: Enhanced Mindset

Along with gaining an enhanced body, you might also gain an enhanced *mindset* — specifically, a mindset having a greater number of success-creating mind elements, or perspectives, feelings, and mind-habits that promote success.

2nd Possible Benefit: Enhanced Self-image

You might gain an enhanced, or more beneficial, self-image. And, along with that, enhanced self-confidence and self-esteem.

3rd Possible Benefit: Success-creation Knowledge

You might gain powerful new success-driving knowledge. While on your weight success journey you might discover, or re-confirm, that most or all of the 19 success drivers that are propelling you to success in your weight success journey can also be used to expedite success in *any other significant endeavor of your life*.

4th Possible Benefit: Mind Awareness

You might discover, or at least become more aware of, the presence, power, and performance of your subconscious mind. And, you might learn of several processes for deliberately communicating with your subconscious mind, thereby giving you the means for deliberately enlisting the performance of your subconscious mind for achieving certain worthwhile ends, any time you desire to do so.

5th Possible Benefit: Daily Good Feeling

You might realize that your weight success journey isn't just some exercise in counting calories and eating certain foods. You might discover that it's actually a special, outstanding accomplishment — an accomplishment worthy of daily recognition and applause, and something you should allow yourself to derive a good feeling from — *every day*.

6th Possible Benefit: Expanded Life Journey

Keep this in mind. Your weight success journey is part of a larger journey, a journey in lifelong personal achievement and fulfillment. As such, you might discover that by succeeding at your weight success journey you're expanding your life journey into something even more beneficial and fulfilling than you previously imagined. This was discussed in the *How the Weight Success Method Enhances Your Life Journey* chapter (p. **157**).

Opportunity to Help Others Have a Better Life

Many people cling to the notion that their life impacts only them. Holding this assumption enables them to rationalize that it doesn't matter what they do, or how they live, or what kind of person they decide to be.

But they're wrong. Each person's life *does* impact the life of others — in particular those closest to them, such as parents, spouse, children, grandchildren, siblings, friends, neighbors. Whenever we do something that amounts to us becoming a finer person or creating a more beneficial life it *positively* impacts the lives of those close to us. Conversely, whenever we do something that amounts to us becoming a less-fine person or living a less beneficial life it *negatively* impacts the lives of those close to us. These two things happen regardless of whether we know they're happening and also regardless of whether we want them to happen.

What's more, the impact of some things we do extends beyond us. By a cause-and-effect chain this impact ultimately extends to people we've never met, even to those not yet born.

So how does this pertain to healthy-weight living? In two ways. First, when we make the decision to live the rest of our life in our healthy-weight range, our life becomes a powerful role model for healthy-weight living — a role model that some of those near and dear to us will ultimately emulate. Second, when we live the latter years of our life in our healthy-weight range we reduce the likelihood of contracting a debilitating condition resulting from extended overweight living.

So as a result, two major positive outcomes occur. First, by being a role model for healthy-weight living you (a) inspire and help others to do the same, which (b) makes their life even better, and also (c) makes the world even better, and finally (d) makes your life even more meaningful and beneficial. Second, by reducing the chance of contracting a debilitating condition from overweight living you reduce the chance of someone close to you having to carry the burden of looking after you or taking care of you for years while you're living in an incapacitated state.

8th Possible Benefit:
Life Enhancement from Getting Input from God

You might discover and apply throughout your life a simple method for gaining insights from God — these insights enabling you to more readily solve stubborn problems and achieve challenging goals (this method being the Three Steps to Getting and Using Input from God, page **117**).

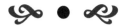

Contrary to what most people assume, the potential benefits of pursuing and creating lifelong Healthy-weight Living are manifold. Done the right way, it can be one of life's simplest pleasures and also most gratifying accomplishments.

CHAPTER 25: Why Most Persons Never Pursue Weight Control

MOST PERSONS hold numerous misconceptions pertaining to healthy-weight living. These misconceptions cause the majority of people to never make a whole-hearted attempt at creating it. Here are nine common misconceptions that cause people to avoid pursuing healthy-weight living.

Misconception 1: Healthy-weight living is an end-result one must achieve. *The Reality:* Healthy-weight living is an ongoing success-creation process that one sustains by doing simple weight success actions each day.

Misconception 2: Healthy-weight living is a far-off situation. *The Reality:* For most persons it can be attained in a matter of just a few months. Or, if one is a lot overweight, it can be attained in a year or so, which although slightly longer is still a relatively short time.

Misconception 3: Healthy-weight living is hard to accomplish. *The Reality:* If one applies a certain method — namely, the Weight Success Method — healthy-weight living is relatively easy to attain, or at least much easier than most persons imagine.

Misconception 4: Maintaining healthy-weight living is joyless, limiting drudgery that involves much sacrifice. *The Reality:* When pursued a certain way (using the Weight Success Method) healthy-weight living brings more enjoyment, happiness, freedom, and gratification than most persons imagine.

Misconception 5: Certain fat-promoting factors can subvert or prevent healthy-weight living. *The Reality:* There's not a single fat-promoting factor that can prevent a person from creating healthy-weight living.

Misconception 6: Creating healthy-weight living requires special medicine or medical procedure. *The Reality:* Although a medical procedure might be a helpful aid for creating healthy-weight living for a few people, it's likely not a requirement for anyone to create healthy-weight living success.

Misconception 7: Creating healthy-weight living requires daily exercise. *The Reality:* Although exercise can be helpful and beneficial, it's not a requirement for succeeding at creating healthy-weight living for anyone.

Misconception 8: Creating healthy-weight living requires applying a strict dietary regimen or a particular dietary program. *The Reality:* It usually helps to apply a preferred dietary program that fits one's personal preferences, needs, and lifestyle, but there's no one specific dietary program that's a requirement for creating healthy-weight living.

Misconception 9: After healthy-weight living is achieved, it doesn't last for long. *The Reality:* It's true that for the past fifty years or so most persons who have lost weight, or achieved a certain weight goal, have eventually gained back the weight they lost. But, this has happened because most persons haven't applied a method for *maintaining* healthy-weight living once they've achieved it. This book changes that. By applying the Weight Success Method you stay living in your healthy-weight range the rest of your life ... and it likely happens easily and enjoyably, or at least more easily and enjoyably than you likely imagine it to be.

Summation

Misconceptions pertaining to healthy-weight living prevent most persons from ever striving to achieve it, and also work to defeat those persons who do attempt it.

Nine Main Misconceptions Pertaining to Healthy-weight Living are:

1 – It's an end-result that one achieves (as opposed to an activity that one sustains).

2 – It's a far-off situation.

3 – It's hard to accomplish.

4 – Maintaining it involves joyless drudgery and much sacrifice.

5 – Certain fat-promoting factors can subvert or prevent it.

6 – Achieving it requires special medicine or medical procedure.

7 – Achieving it requires daily exercise.

8 – Achieving it requires applying a strict dietary regimen or a particular dietary program.

9 – Once it's achieved it won't last for long.

> For more on misconceptions and false assumptions that are sabotaging weight management, go to the *16 False Assumptions that are Sabotaging Us* chapter (p. **146**) and also *Special Extra Section: Why Most Persons Aren't Pursuing Weight Management* (p. **8**).

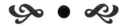

Once humankind understands what healthy-weight living really is and the easiest way to create it, the growing global overweightness trend will <u>stop</u> and worldwide healthy-weight living will <u>ascend</u>.

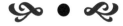

Do
Weight Success Actions
<u>EVERY DAY</u>

CHAPTER 26: Message from Healthy-weight Living

Throughout this book, I (the author) have done the talking. So, for some personification fun I'm bringing in *Healthy-weight Living* itself to impart a special message.

Hello, **I** am Healthy-weight living!

You might think you know me.
> *But most likely you do <u>not</u> know me. I'll explain.*

You think I'm far away and out of reach.
> *But I'm near you this very moment.*

You think I'm hard to get.
> *But I'm so easy to have you don't believe it.*

You think I'm no fun.
> *But I bring more benefits, enjoyment, and gratification than you imagine.*

You think I'm an <u>achievement</u> — a destination or end-result that you arrive at.
> *But, actually, I'm a <u>process</u> — an ongoing **success-creation process** you do each day.*

You think I can be killed by certain fat-promoting factors.
> *But not a one can stop me, not a one can prevent me.*

You think I exist to harass, punish, and limit you.
> *But, in truth, I exist to help you live an easier, happier, freer life.*

You think the way you entice me into your life is to change the way you EAT.
> *But, actually, the way you cause me to join you is to change the way you THINK — in particular, the way you think about your self, your mind, your life, weight management, and <u>me</u> — Healthy-weight Living.*

You think that for me to stick with you you need a special medicine or medical procedure.
> *But — even though a medical procedure might be helpful for some — I don't absolutely require it.*

You think it's required that you exercise each day in order for me to be your friend.
> *But — even though exercise can be helpful and beneficial — I don't require it of anyone.*

You think it's required that you embrace a strict dietary regimen in order for me to accept you.
> *But I don't require that.*

You think it's required that you work hard and sacrifice in order for me to stick around.
> *But I don't require that.*

You think I'm fickle and fleeting.
> *But I'm not. I'll happily stay with you <u>forever</u> IF you treat me a certain way. All I request is that you truly want me to be with you, that you view me in a positive light, that you honor me each day with some whole-mind attention, and that you pursue me as a **daily success-creation process**.*

Yes, I am Healthy-weight living. Know me for what I <u>really</u> am; know how I <u>really</u> work. Then I will become one of your closest, most loyal friends — for life. And, once you and I become friends, please tell your other friends about me. Because I would like to someday be their friend, too. Truth is, I'd like to be a friend of everyone on the planet. But that's not likely to happen today, because most people are confused about me. They think they know who I am and how I work.
> *But, actually, they do not. And, as long as they don't know how I really work, they will be avoiding me, and will be refraining from inviting me into their life.*

Still, it brings me great comfort to realize that YOU now know the truth about me. I trust you'll be putting it to good use ... for the rest of your life.

Most people who aren't pursuing healthy-weight living are doing so because they're holding an erroneous conception of healthy-weight living. Amazingly, most people don't know how healthy-weight living works.

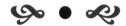

LIFELONG WEIGHT SUCCESS DYNAMIC

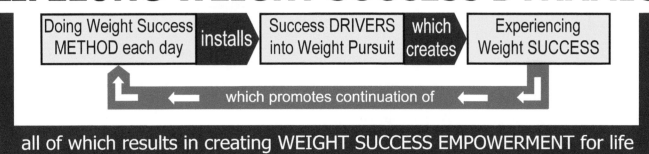

Doing Weight Success METHOD each day **installs** Success DRIVERS into Weight Pursuit **which creates** Experiencing Weight SUCCESS

which promotes continuation of

all of which results in creating WEIGHT SUCCESS EMPOWERMENT for life

WEIGHT SUCCESS = Living most or all of one's days in one's desired healthy-weight range <u>and</u> deriving benefits, enjoyment, and fulfillment from it. ~ For description of benefits created by weight success, see Chapter 7 (p. **80**). For description of enjoyment and fulfillment created by doing the Weight Success Method and achieving healthy-weight living, go to Chapter 17 (p. **123**), Chapter 22 (p. **157**), and Chapter 24 (p. **168**). ~ A person who's in process of creating weight success we call a *Weight Winner.*

CHAPTER 27: Handy Extra Tools for Even Easier Healthy-weight Creation

To create a handy printout of this chapter, go to: correllconcepts.com/toolkit.pdf

DOING THE five Daily Actions of the Weight Success Method is enough to create healthy-weight living success. But you might find that using one or more of these optional tools can make it even faster, easier, or more enjoyable. A big key to succeeding at important pursuits, or achieving important goals, is to recognize daily progress. To do this it helps to *measure and record* progress on a daily basis. This chapter provides three optional tools you can use for accomplishing that: the Weight Success Actions Scorecard, the Win-Day Calendar, and the Weight-reduction Success Graph. The Scorecard and the Calendar can be used in both weight maintenance pursuit and weight reduction pursuit. The Weight-reduction Success Graph is designed for use only in weight reduction pursuit. We'll examine each.

1 – Weight Success Actions Scorecard

Are you one who likes keeping score? Many people enjoy recording their activities and breaking personal best records. If you happen to be such a person, this optional tool is for you. To help you "score" your daily Weight Success Actions and accomplishments we're providing the *Weight Success Actions Scorecard* shown on page **175**. If you like, make copies of it for your personal use. It's designed to record up to fourteen days.

You'll note that with the Scorecard you can score daily points for doing the five Daily Actions of the Weight Success Method, described in Chapter 2 (p. **44**), and also for doing optional actions described in the *Six More Mind Motivators* chapter (p. **110**).

You'll also note that higher daily point total indicates greater activity; lower total indicates lesser activity. This enables you to compare one day to another. So, if you like, you can track your daily personal Weight Success Actions.

> NOTE: The point amounts were arbitrarily set by the writer. They don't correlate with any scientific study. If you disagree with the point amounts shown, just change them to whatever you feel best fits your situation.

2 – Win-Day Calendar

Get a calendar that shows individual days for each month, the kind you can hang on a wall or set up on a desk or dresser. Put it where you'll see it each day.

For each day that your daily weight reading is a *desired* reading, write a big "W" in that day. The "W" stands for *WIN* or *Winning Day*. It indicates that you were a healthy-weight Winner on that day. An example of how the W's might look on the calendar is shown on page **176**.

And, each week that you score at least six "W's" you can call that a healthy-weight success week. And, each month that you score at least four healthy-weight success weeks you can call that a healthy-weight success month.

Challenge yourself to see how long a string of "W's" you can get. Pretty soon you'll be filling an entire month with "W's". And eventually you'll be having strings of months with all "W's".

And remember, each day that you write that "W" on the calendar, generate a happy, positive feeling. It means, you're a WINNER — specifically, a Healthy-weight Winner. Being a Healthy-weight Winner on any particular day is a *noteworthy* accomplishment. Feel *good* about it — each day.

3 – Weight-reduction Success Graph

If you happen to be in weight reduction mode, use the graph on page **178** to record your daily progress. This can be very motivating. For an example of how it looks filled in, see page **179**.

Weight Success Actions Scorecard™ | Daily Point Calculator

	DATE→												
FIVE DAILY ACTIONS of the Weight Success Method (described in Ch. 2)													
Did Daily Action 1–Weighing (p. 44) | **50** pts.													
Got a Desired Weight Reading | **100** pts.													
Did Daily Action 2A–Reinforcement (p. 45) **or** Daily Action 2B–Correction (p. 48) | **50** pts.													
Did Daily Action 3–Benefits Directive (p. 50) | **50** pts.													
Did Daily Action 4–Goal Statement (p. 54) | **50** pts.													
Did extra Goal Statement iterations for Daily Action 4 | Score **1** point for each one over 25													
Did Daily Action 5–Guided Eating (p. 56) | **50** pts.													
(A) TOTAL POINTS for doing Daily Actions													
OPTIONAL ACTIONS													
Did my daily exercise | **100** pts.													
Did at least three of the eight eating actions described in Ch. 12 (p. 102) | **30** pts.													
Did Motivator 2: Backup Depiction Statement – Ch. 13 (p. 110) | Score **1** point per iteration													
Did Motivator 3: Upcoming-day Description – Ch. 13 (p. 112) | **30** pts.													
Did Motivator 4: Day-end Thanks – Ch. 13 (p. 114) | **30** pts.													
Did Motivator 5: Benefits Visualization – Ch. 13 (p. 114) | **30** pts.													
Did Motivator 6: Goal Reminders – Ch. 13 (p. 115) | **30** pts													
Applied my preferred dietary program (or did right eating) for the entire day | **100** pts.													
Thanked God for the opportunity to be alive & the power to live my healthy weight | **100** pts.													
Did the setback-reversal process, if needed – Ch. 10 (p. 88) | **100** pts.													
(B) TOTAL POINTS for Optional Actions													
GRAND TOTAL POINTS for the Day (A + B)													

INSTRUCTIONS: In the line near the top, put the date of the day being scored. In the boxes beneath that date, insert the number of points you achieved from doing each of the Actions (both Daily Actions and Optional Actions). Then add up the TOTAL points for the Daily Actions (A) and the TOTAL points for the Optional Actions (B). Finally, add those two totals together for the GRAND TOTAL number of points you achieved for the day. ~ To easily print out this chart, go to: **correllconcepts.com/toolkit.pdf**

Example of Partial Win-Day Calendar with Some W's Filled In

SUN	MON	TUE	WED	THU	FRI	SAT
1 W	*2* W	*3* W	*4* W	*5* W	*6* W	*7* W
8 W	*9* W	*10* W	*11* W	*12*	*13*	*14*
15	*16*	*17*	*18*	*19*	*20*	*21*

Note: The above graphic was designed to illustrate the W's, which is why there's only a partial month shown.

If you like, also record your daily weight (scale reading) number on the calendar. Write it in the lower right corner of the square for each day.

Making Your Own Calendar

In case you might prefer to make your own calendar instead of buying one, on the next page (**177**) is a blank calendar sheet you can use for any month. Print copies of it for your use. For each month, fill in the appropriate squares with the appropriate date number for each day. Put the date in the upper left corner of the square. Then use the sheet to record your winning days with a "W."

Win-Day Calendar™

Month of:					Year:	
SUN	**MON**	**TUE**	**WED**	**THU**	**FRI**	**SAT**

INSTRUCTIONS: Make copies for your use. Fill in the month and year in the line at the top. In the upper left corner of each day box that pertains to that particular month, write in the date of that day. Each day that your daily weight reading is a *desired* reading, write a big "W" in the box. Also, if you like, write in the scale weight reading you got for that day (suggested that you put it in the lower right corner of the box). ~ To easily print out this chart, go to: **correllconcepts.com/toolkit.pdf**

Weight-reduction Success Graph™

Month of: _____   Year: _____

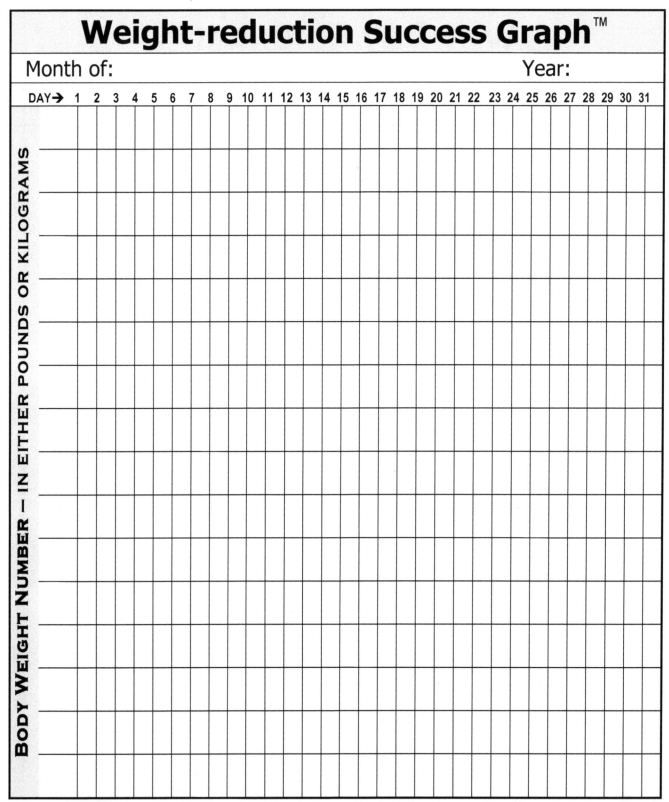

INSTRUCTIONS: If you happen to presently be in <u>weight-reduction</u> mode, make copies of this graph to record your daily progress. For each month, put your projected declining weight numbers along the left side of the graph. Fill in the month and year at the top. ~ On the next page (**179**) is an example to illustrate how it would work. It's filled in with example pound weight numbers (shown in green) and an example graph line showing a person's body weight for 31 days of that month (in red). ~ To easily print out this graph, go to: **correllconcepts.com/toolkit.pdf**

Weight-reduction Success Graph™

Month of: *AUGUST*   Year: *2018*

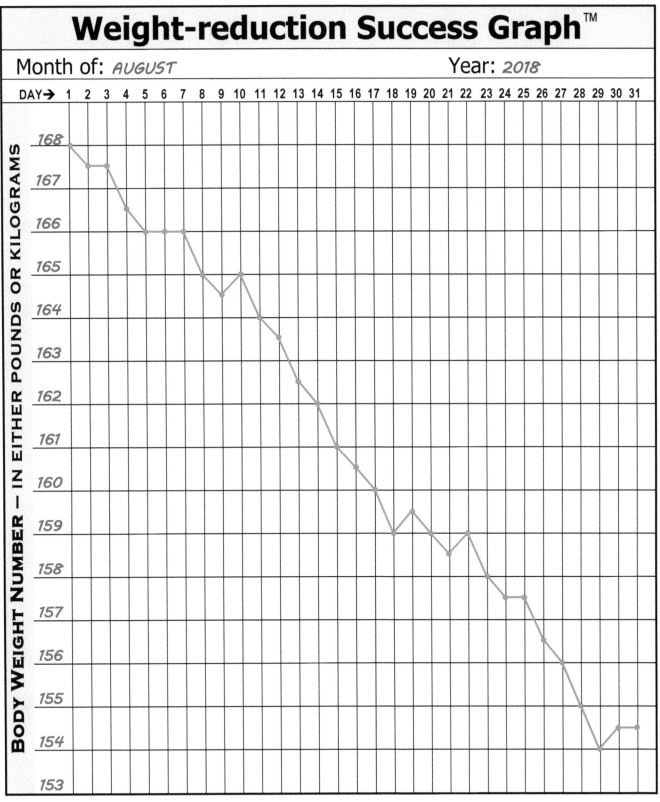

EXAMPLE: At the top, fill in the month and year (shown in blue). Fill in the target weight numbers (shown in green). If you weigh in kilograms (as opposed to pounds), it's recommended that your weight numbers be in half-kilogram increments. So, for example, if your present weight were, say, 76 kilograms, the declining weight increments would be: 76, 75.5, 75, 74.5, 74, 73.5, 73 … and so on. If a day's weight turns out to be half way between two weight numbers, then position the dot for that day (shown in red) half way between the two numbers, as done for some days in the above graph.

Many people fail to create healthy-weight living <u>not</u> because they don't know what to do and <u>not</u> because they don't want to do it but, rather, because they *forget* to do it.

Since eating is a daily activity it means that creating healthy-weight living must also be a *daily* activity. The easiest, most effective daily activity for creating healthy-weight living is doing the five daily actions (p. 44) of the Weight Success Method each day.

I know this might sound unbelievable, but a main thing that will stop you from realizing lifelong healthy-weight living is failing to remember to do all five daily actions each day. So, I suggest you set up a fail-proof reminder mechanism that will remind you each day to do these five actions. Here's a sample way to do it.

Print out one or more copies of the rectangle-enclosed messages on the next page (p. **181**). If you need different sizes than these, just put a copy on a copier machine, enlarge or reduce the image to suit your needs, and then print it.

Place copies where you'll see them every day. Possibilities include: (a) in your bedroom, (b) on the refrigerator, (c) in your wallet or purse, (d) in your car, (e) on your computer, and (f) on your exercise equipment.

Plus, also put digital messages on your computer screen, smartphone, and other devices you access every day. For that, go to:

http://correllconcepts.com/wfm-jpg.htm

In short, do whatever it takes to set up a fail-proof reminder system that will remind you each day to do the five daily actions of the Weight Success Method. Installing a daily reminder mechanism is a vital key to more easily living the rest of your life in your healthy-weight range.

> It may be that more instances of failure result from **forgetting** to do what one should be doing than from **not knowing** what one should do.

Weight Success Method

Do it every day. Takes less than eight minutes.
1 – Weighing
2 – Reinforcement or Correction
3 – Benefits Directive
4 – Goal Statement
5 – Guided Eating
(plus Daily Exercise Activity)

Weight Success Method

Do it every day. Takes less than eight minutes.
1 – Weighing
2 – Reinforcement or Correction
3 – Benefits Directive
4 – Goal Statement
5 – Guided Eating
(plus Daily Exercise Activity)

Weight Success Method

Do it every day. Takes less than eight minutes.
1 – Weighing
2 – Reinforcement or Correction
3 – Benefits Directive
4 – Goal Statement
5 – Guided Eating
(plus Daily Exercise Activity)

INSTRUCTIONS: Make one or more copies of this page. If you need different sizes than these, just put a copy on a copier machine, enlarge or reduce the image to suit your needs, and then print it. Cut out the reminder messages and place them where you'll see them every day. ~ To easily print out this page, go to: **correllconcepts.com/toolkit.pdf**

SECTION C:
GOING NATIONWIDE

— A How-to Guide for Creating Nationwide Weight Success —

THIS SECTION describes a program that I believe would be the easiest, most effective way to guide the citizenry of a nation to weight success — a.k.a. healthy-weight living. For future reference this program is dubbed *Nationwide Weight Success Initiative,* or NWSI for short.

We define *weight success* as: Living most or all of one's days in one's desired healthy-weight range <u>and</u> deriving benefits, enjoyment, and fulfillment from it. The ultimate goal of the Nationwide Weight Success Initiative is to have nearly everyone in the nation engaged in weight success — or living most or all of their days in their desired healthy-weight range and deriving benefits, enjoyment, and fulfillment from it.

To be effective, any program that aims to motivate an entire nation to pursue healthy-weight living should — or perhaps *must* — include the following eight actions:

1. Identify the misconceptions that exist regarding weight management, right eating, and healthy-weight living;

2. Refute and dispel those misconceptions;

3. Replace the dispelled misconceptions with healthy-weight-promoting conceptions;

4. Describe the possible benefits people can derive from weight success;

5. Explain that the key to creating healthy-weight living is to do Weight Success Actions *every day* — both during pursuit of weight reduction <u>and</u> during pursuit of weight maintenance;

6. Equip people with the wherewithal, including a simple step-by-step weight success program, that makes it easy for them to do Weight Success Actions every day;

7. Provide proof that anyone can easily succeed at healthy-weight living;

8. Make healthy-weight living appear to be, and to actually be, *more rewarding* than non-healthy-weight living, as viewed by the citizenry of the nation.

The above eight actions might not be the only actions that can contribute to creating nationwide healthy-weight living. But they're the essential ones needed for it. I'll now explain each.

ACTION 1: Identify Misconceptions

The starting point to motivating the people of a nation to pursue living their life in their healthy-weight range is to identify the many misconceptions that exist regarding weight management, right eating, and living in one's healthy-weight range. This likely will require broad interviewing and perhaps some psycho-analytical research. Here's the situation.

Most people are carrying in their mind a mountain of weight management misconceptions — including rationalization, self-delusion, and erroneous beliefs. These misconceptions are preventing them from pursuing, or from even considering pursuing, right eating and healthy-weight living. And, for those commendable few who do decide to "give it a try," these misconceptions eventually sabotage their every initiative at doing healthy-weight living, thereby dooming them to being a perpetual yo-yo dieter.

For a starting point in identifying these misconceptions I would suggest referring to (a) the 16 false assumptions listed in the *16 False Assumptions that Are Sabotaging Us* chapter (p. **146**) and also (b) the nine misconceptions described in the *Why*

Most Persons Never Pursue Weight Control chapter (p. **170**).

ACTION 2: Refute the Misconceptions

The second action is to line up all the misconceptions — that is, rationalizations, self-delusions, and false assumptions — and shoot 'em dead with refutation. And, then periodically shoot 'em again. This is a situation where beating a dead horse is a *good* thing to be doing, because the horse of weight management misconceptions is big, powerful, and pervasive, and could resurrect any time the refutation stops for long.

This Action Two, and the actions to follow, should be done via a powerful, captivating, broad-based *ongoing* nationwide advertising–communications–publicity campaign constructed to inspire and equip every individual to pursue and create weight success. For future reference I call this campaign the *Weight Success Communication Campaign*.

ACTION 3: Install Healthy-weight-promoting Conceptions

The third action, which would be concurrent with Action Two, is to present the "opposites" of the discredited misconceptions. Or, put another way, in this Action Three we replace the counterproductive rationalizations, self-delusions, and erroneous beliefs — which have been preventing most people from pursuing and succeeding at healthy-weight living — with productive perspectives and beliefs that promote, inspire, and sustain the pursuit and creation of healthy-weight living. This action won't be a one-time occurrence but, instead, along with Action Two, will be ongoing for many years. It would be performed through every communication vehicle available, including the media used in the Weight Success Communication Campaign.

ACTION 4: Describe Weight Success Benefits

The fourth action, which would be concurrent with Action Three, is to describe the many good things that a person can derive from right eating and healthy-weight living — which we call *weight success benefits*. Then, through the Weight Success Communication Campaign, urge each person to identify those benefits that apply specifically to them and their situation. In doing this it's likely that the weight success benefit that will, or should, receive top billing will be: Maximizing the chance of *living healthier longer* — or maximizing the chance of living free of certain debilitating illnesses and body malfunctions.

ACTION 5: Explain the Key to Healthy-weight Living

The fifth action is to communicate to the entire nation that the key to easier healthy-weight living is: Do Weight Success Actions *every day* — both in the weight-reduction phase and in the weight-maintenance phase. Explain that this can be accomplished by doing the actions prescribed in the Weight Success Method, which causes success drivers to be included in one's weight success pursuit. (An explanation of success drivers is provided in the Success Drivers section, page **23**.) And also, communicate to the nation the *Lifelong Weight Success Dynamic* (p. **61**).

ACTION 6: Equip People with the Tools for Easily Doing Weight Success Actions Every Day

The sixth action, which would be concurrent with Action Five, is to equip each person — meaning, the entire nation — with the essential wherewithal they need for easily doing Weight Success Actions every day.

The following six tools, or resources, constitute the essential wherewithal that most persons need in order to easily do Weight Success Actions every day.

Tool 1: A step-by-step healthy-weight living program — a.k.a. weight success methodology — that makes it easy for them to do Weight Success Actions every day — both during weight reduction and during weight maintenance. A recommended program would be the Weight Success Method. All this could be provided on a website set up by the Nationwide Weight Success Initiative, and also made available via a paperback booklet and other media forms.

Tool 2: An accurate bathroom scale, or daily access to one. Instructions on obtaining a good scale could be provided on a website set up by the Nationwide Weight Success Initiative. Go to the *Weighing and Scale Info* chapter (p. **82**) for details on scales.

Tool 3: Knowledge of one's healthy-weight range. A means for easy automatic ascertainment of one's healthy-weight range could be provided on a website set up by the Nationwide Weight Success Initiative. Also, we must make it possible for a person to make a phone call (in place of accessing a website), give their height, age, gender, and body type information, and receive back their healthy-weight range. This could be handled automatically, as opposed to having an actual person receiving the call. Go to the *Healthy-weight Range in Detail* chapter (p. **76**) for details on healthy-weight range.

Tool 4: Recognition of one's weight success benefits — that is, awareness of the benefits that a person will derive from living in their healthy-weight range. A listing of generic weight success benefits could be provided on a website set up by the Nationwide Weight Success Initiative. Go to the *Weight Success Benefits in Detail* chapter (p. **80**) for details on weight success benefits.

Tool 5: Selection of a dietary program or eating strategy, which could be either an established bona fide dietary program already on the market or a program of a person's own design. This program would be applied in conjunction with the recommended Healthy-weight Living program (Tool 1 above). A sample listing of the many available die-

tary program choices could be provided on a website set up by the Nationwide Weight Success Initiative. Go to Startup Action 7 (p. **40**) for details on preferred dietary program.

Tool 6: A weight success mindset — that is, a set of perspectives that promotes doing right eating and living in one's healthy-weight range. A description of a sample recommended mindset could be provided on a website set up by the Nationwide Weight Success Initiative. Go to Startup Action 5 (p. **37**) for details on weight success mindset.

So, these six resources, or instructions on how to get them, could be provided by the Nationwide Weight Success Initiative via website and also other media.

ACTION 7: Provide Proof that Healthy-weight Living Is Easily Doable

The seventh action is to provide proof that anyone can succeed at living in their healthy-weight range if (a) they make the decision to do so and (b) they get their whole mind involved in the act, which can be accomplished by applying the recommended Healthy-weight Living program (Tool 1 above), and (c) they pursue weight management as a process of doing Weight Success Actions every day.

There are many ways this proof can be provided. One way is to provide explanation of *why* the recommended weight-management method works. (Such an explanation exists in the Why the Weight Success Method Gets Your Whole Mind Involved chapter, page **129**.)

Another way, which likely would be the most convincing, is to provide examples. And, one of the most powerful examples is *demonstration by leaders.* In the case of government-created programs, such as the Nationwide Weight Success Initiative, the leaders are those persons chosen to lead and manage the nation. In the case of the United States, this leadership comprises the key, or high-ranking, persons working in the administration and congressional branches of our government.

So, the most convincing proof that anyone can and should succeed at living in their healthy-weight range would be for the president and his cabinet and also all the senators and representatives of congress to apply the program set forth in the Weight Success Method and, thereby, succeed at living in their healthy-weight range.

This action would be compelling evidence that what the Nationwide Weight Success Initiative is telling the entire nation it should be doing is, in fact, doable, effective, and desirable. Or, put another way, if the several hundred persons who constitute our national leadership do it, then it would be clearly obvious to the entire country that (a) *anyone* can do it and (b) everyone *should be* doing it.

Conversely, if the country's leadership isn't doing what it's telling the citizenry of the nation it should be doing — which is, living in one's healthy-weight range — this would cause many persons to conclude that our leaders are being dishonest and hypocritical. Which would be a significant hindrance to maximizing the success of the Nationwide Weight Success Initiative.

ACTION 8: Make Healthy-weight Living Appear to Be More Rewarding than Non-healthy-weight Living

The eighth action is: *Make people realize that healthy-weight living is* more rewarding *than non-healthy-weight living.* When people view healthy-weight living as being more rewarding (enjoyable, gratifying) than non-healthy-weight living, they choose to pursue healthy-weight living. Conversely, when they view non-healthy-weight living as being more rewarding than healthy-weight living, they choose to pursue non-healthy-weight living.

So, a main aim of the Weight Success Communication Campaign should be to make doing healthy-weight living appear to be, and to actually be, more rewarding than doing non-healthy-weight living, as viewed by the citizenry of the nation. By doing this we motivate people to pursue healthy-weight living and to forego non-healthy-weight living. Expressed in greater detail, this is how we could do it.

Every type of performance, including right eating performance and wrong eating performance, has both an upside and a downside. The upside is whatever a person likes about doing the particular performance. The downside is whatever the person dislikes about doing it. So, the net reward of any particular performance is "the upside minus the downside."

Which means, to expand the net reward that a person derives from doing healthy-weight living we must (a) expand the upside and (b) diminish the downside of doing healthy-weight living, as viewed by the performer. Conversely, to diminish the net reward that a person derives from doing non-healthy-weight living we must (a) expand the downside and (b) diminish the upside of doing non-healthy-weight living, as viewed by the performer.

What all this comes down to is, the Weight Success Communication Campaign should include messages and programs designed to accomplish these four results.

1. *EXPAND the* upside *of right eating and healthy-weight living.* ❧ Identify the full upside picture of right eating and healthy-weight living and then project this picture into the minds of the nation.

> NOTE: For a full description of the upside to weight success, see these four chapters: Chapter 7 (p. **80**), Chapter 17 (p. **123**), Chapter 22 (p. **157**), and Chapter 24 (p. **168**).

2. *DIMINISH the* downside *of right eating.* ❧ Identify the aspects of right eating that some people might view as downside and then help them realize that these aspects can be diminished to insignificance. (Note: Part of what the recommended Weight Success Method does is help people reduce to insignificance the imagined downside of right eating.)

3. *EXPAND the* downside *of wrong eating and non-healthy-weight living.* ❧ Identify the full downside picture of wrong eating and non-healthy-weight living and then project this picture into the minds of the nation.

4. *DIMINISH the* upside *of wrong eating.* ❧ Identify those aspects of wrong eating, or overeating, that some people might view as upside and then help them realize that these aspects bring large unintended bad consequences.

These four results can be summed up by this infographic.

In the MIND of the citizenry:

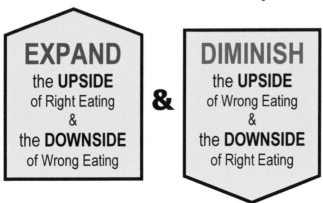

Conclusion

The most effective way to cause the citizenry of a nation to achieve weight success is to implement a national program that motivates and equips people to do vital weight success actions every day — both while in weight reduction phase and while in weight maintenance phase. The extent to which a program accomplishes this will be the extent to which a nation succeeds in creating nationwide healthy-weight living.

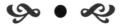

SUMMING UP
For Nationwide Weight Success:

1. Identify misconceptions.

2. Refute misconceptions.

3. Install healthy-weight-promoting conceptions.

4. Describe weight success benefits.

5. Explain the key to healthy-weight living.

6. Equip people with the tools for easily doing Weight Success Actions every day.

7. Provide proof that healthy-weight living is easily doable.

8. Make healthy-weight living appear to be, and to actually be, more rewarding than non-healthy-weight living.

If we as a nation do those eight actions overweight living will decline and healthy-weight living will ascend. Or, put another way, most of the people in the nation will achieve lifelong *weight success* — that is, they will live most or all of their days in their desired healthy-weight range and derive benefits, enjoyment, and fulfillment from it.

SECTION D:
GLOSSARY OF TERMS

The Lexicon of Weight Success

Accomplishment: A desired situation, or goal, that has been realized

Achievement (a.k.a. achieving): The act of creating a certain desired situation, or the act of achieving a certain goal

Achievement Action (a.k.a. achieving action): An action that contributes to achieving a certain desired situation or goal

Achievement Activity (a.k.a. achieving activity): An activity that contributes to achieving a certain desired situation or goal

Achievement Pursuit: A pursuit that's conceived and executed in a way that involves performing ongoing achievement actions, or performing actions that foster achievement of a certain desired situation or goal

Achieving (a.k.a. achievement): The act of creating a certain desired situation, or the act of achieving a certain goal

Acting As-if: (1) The act of holding in mind an assumption that a particular situation presently exists or is in the process of coming about, and then conducting one's thinking, feelings, and actions in accordance with that assumption. (2) A real-life role-play of a situation one wants to exist or have happen.

Actualization (a.k.a. actualizing, actualization process): The act of creating an _actual_ situation that corresponds to a certain _imagined_ situation, such as a goal

Automatic Eating: (See Unguided Eating)

Belief: Assumption

Believing: The act of assuming that a particular situation exists

Calorie (a.k.a. food calorie): A measure of energy that a food or beverage provides. Note: In this book when the term _calorie_ is used it's referring to "metabolizable calories," or calories that the human body is capable of metabolizing, or converting into energy.

Causal-factor Eradication: An approach to creating life enhancement that involves eradicating a particular factor that's causing a problem at the present time

C-B-A Process: A three-step process consisting of Communicating, Believing, and Appreciating. It's a key process of the Weight Success Method, specifically used in the Guided Eating Process of Daily Action 5.

Daily Achievement Action (a.k.a. daily success action): (1) An action that's performed every day or most days for the duration of a particular pursuit, and which contributes to achieving a certain desired situation or goal.

Daily Reminder Mechanism: Any tool or means used for reminding you each day to do the five daily actions of the Weight Success Method

Daily Success Action (a.k.a. daily winning action): A success action that's performed every day or most days for the duration of a particular life-enhancing pursuit

Daily Weighing Hour: The set 60-minute period in which you weigh yourself each day

Daily Weight Success Action: A weight success action that's performed every day or most days for the duration of a weight success pursuit

Depiction Statement (a.k.a. verbal depiction): A verbal or word description of a situation. Typically the situation being depicted is either (a) an imagined desired situation you want to actualize, or make real or (b) a desirable present situation you want to perpetuate. The Healthy-weight Goal Statement is the primary depiction statement used in the Weight Success Method. Optional backup depiction statements are also verbal depiction statements.

Desired Weight Reading: (a) When in weight <u>reduction</u> pursuit, a desired weight reading would be a scale reading that shows a weight <u>loss</u> from the prior day. (b) When in weight <u>maintenance</u> pursuit, a desired weight reading would be any scale reading that's <u>within</u> your healthy-weight range

Directive: An instruction, order, or request delivered to your mind for the purpose of motivating it to perform a certain action or create a certain result

Don't-eat-it Signal: (See Stop-eating Signal)

During-eating Self-talk: Guided-eating self-talk that's delivered while *in the process* of eating

Easiest Way to Realize Healthy-weight Living: The Weight Success Method, which makes each day be a Weight Success Day

Eating: The act of consuming food, including liquid food (a.k.a. beverage)

Fat-promoting Factors: Factors that promote overeating or fat gain, or make it easier for a person to overeat or gain weight (but which do *not cause* overeating or fat gain)

Food: Any solid or liquid nutritive substance consumed by humans

Full-stomach Feeling: A feeling that your stomach is filled with food. It typically includes a feeling of pressure or tightening at the top of your stomach, or where your stomach joins your throat.

This feeling can come even when your stomach isn't completely full.

Goal-achieving Action (a.k.a. achieving action): An action that contributes to achieving a certain goal

Goal-achieving Day: A day in which one does certain goal-achieving actions. In one's weight success pursuit, a goal-achieving day is sometimes called a Weight Success Day

Goal-promoting Belief: A belief that promotes actualization of a certain goal

Goal-promoting Communication: A communication that tells your mind what it should be doing in way of assisting with achieving a certain goal

Goal-realization Action: A daily action that leads to attainment or realization of a desired situation or goal

Guided Eating (a.k.a. controlled eating, directed eating): Eating activity that's guided by the eater, typically for the purpose of curtailing overeating and, thereby, creating right eating and living at one's desired weight

Guided Eating Process: A three-step process involving Communicating, Believing, and Appreciating, and which is used for creating guided eating

Guided-eating Self-talk: Any message delivered to your self — or your mind — while eating, for the purpose of causing your mind to guide you away from wrong eating and toward right eating, or away from overeating and toward non-overeating

Habit: An automatic frequently-repeated behavior or activity. A habit consists of two components: a physical component and a mental component. The physical component, which we call *action-habit,* is an automatic repeating physical activity. The mental component, which we call *mind-habit,* is an automatic repeating mental process. The mind-habit underlies and drives the action-habit.

Healthy Eating (*a.k.a. healthy-weight eating, right eating*): (1) Eating that promotes good health and living in your healthy-weight range. (2) Eating right foods in right amounts and in a way that creates right eating enjoyment.

Healthy Weight (*a.k.a. right weight*): Every weight that's in your healthy-weight range is regarded as being a healthy weight for you

Healthy-eating Day (*a.k.a. right-eating day*): A day in which your overall eating for the day amounts to right eating and non-overeating

Healthy-weight Achievement Scorecard™ (See Weight Success Actions Scorecard)

Healthy-weight Achievement: The repeated daily act of creating an <u>actual</u> body weight that's within a certain <u>desired</u> healthy-weight range

Healthy-weight Action (*a.k.a. healthy-weight achieving action, healthy-weight-creating action*): (See Weight Success Action)

Healthy-weight Calorie Allotment (*a.k.a. daily calorie allotment*): The amount of daily calories that maintains your body weight within your healthy-weight range

Healthy-weight Daily Method: (See Weight Success Method)

Healthy-weight Eating (*a.k.a. healthy eating, right eating*): (1) Eating that promotes good health and living in your healthy-weight range. (2) Eating right foods in right amounts and in a way that creates right eating enjoyment.

Healthy-weight Eating Actions (*a.k.a. right-eating actions*): Eating actions that result in living in one's healthy-weight range

Healthy-weight Goal Statement (*a.k.a. healthy-weight focus statement*): A word depiction of the ultimate goal, or desired ultimate outcome, of one's weight success endeavor — specifically: *"I am the person of my healthy weight. I am healthy, happy, and doing great."*

Healthy-weight Living Success: (See Weight Success)

Healthy-weight Living: Living most or all of one's days in one's healthy-weight range

Healthy-weight Method: (See Weight Success Method)

Healthy-weight Mindset (*a.k.a. right-eating mindset*): (See Weight Success Mindset)

Healthy-weight Prayer: A prayer expressing thanks to God, including thanks for the opportunity to easily live in one's healthy-weight range

Healthy-weight Range: The weight range that maximizes the likelihood of you living in optimal health. Every weight within your healthy-weight range is regarded as being a healthy weight for you.

Healthy-weight Success: (See Weight Success)

Healthy-weight Success Action: (See Weight Success Action)

Healthy-weight Winner (*a.k.a. weight winner*): A person who's in process of creating weight success

Healthy-Weight Success Day: (See Weight Success Day)

Healthy-weight-creating (*a.k.a. healthy-weight-promoting*): Creating or promoting the creation of healthy-weight living; used, for example, in the context of healthy-weight-creating thoughts, feelings, decisions, actions, communications, foods

Healthy-weight-promoting Action: (See Weight Success Action)

High-power Eat-right Solution: A multi-action procedure for ending recurring overeating and creeping weight gain, used in Optional Action 7 of the setback-reversal process.

Ideal Weight: (1) A body weight that's considered to be ideal for you. (2) A body weight that's most apt to promote good health for you. (3) A body weight number produced by any of the ideal weight formulas that exist in the medical field (ex., the Robinson formula).

Life-enhancing Situation: A new situation that's an improvement over a present situation

Lifelong Weight Success Dynamic: A dynamic in which doing the Weight Success Method each day installs success drivers into one's weight success pursuit which, in turn, results in experiencing weight success which, in turn, fosters continuation of doing the Weight Success Method

Maintenance Achievement: The act of applying success drivers, or success methodology, for the purpose of maintaining a certain situation, or for "staying the same"

Maintenance Eating: Consuming an amount of calories nearly equal to what your body is metabolizing, or "burning up," per day — typically done to maintain yourself in your healthy-weight range

Mealtime Gluttony-eating: (1) Eating until you're stuffed or until your stomach can't hold any more. (2) Overeating at mealtime.

Mind Actions: Actions that occur in one's mind — e.g., thoughts, feelings, and decisions are mind actions

Mind-motivation Action: A daily action that motivates a person to perform the goal-realization actions necessary for attaining or realizing a certain desired situation or goal

New-situation Creation: An approach to creating life enhancement that involves creating a desired *new* situation that, when actualized, automatically replaces a non-desired present situation

Non-healthy Eating (a.k.a. wrong eating, unhealthy eating): Any eating that hinders good health or hinders living in your healthy-weight range — typically, overeating

Open–Insert–Swallow Action (a.k.a. Open–Insert–Swallow Process): The three-action process of opening one's mouth, inserting food into one's mouth, and swallowing the food

Overeating: Consuming more calories than what your body is metabolizing, or "burning up," per day. Note: In this book when the term *calorie* is used it's referring to "metabolizable calories," or calories that the human body is capable of metabolizing, or converting into energy.

Overeating-reversal: The act of replacing recurring overeating and weight gain with right eating and healthy-weight living

Over-snacking: Snacking to the point where it results in overeating for the day

Overweight Body Weight: A body weight that's above your healthy-weight range. An *underweight body weight* would be a weight that's below your healthy-weight range.

Pleasure-priority Eating: Eating that has eating pleasure maximization as its top priority or focus

Preferred Dietary Program (a.k.a. preferred dietary strategy, preferred eating strategy): A set of eating guidelines and eating practices you prefer to follow and which, when followed, cause you to realize good health and healthy-weight living

Preferred Eating Strategy: (See Preferred Dietary Program)

Reinforcement (a.k.a. positive reinforcement): The act of giving someone something they like as a response or consequence for performing a certain action or creating a certain result

Right Amount of Food: (1) An amount of food that promotes living in your healthy-weight range. (2) An amount of food prescribed by your preferred dietary program.

Right Eating (a.k.a. healthy-weight eating, healthy eating): (1) Eating that promotes good health and living in your healthy-weight range. (2) Eating right foods in right amounts and in a way that creates right eating enjoyment. (3) Eating prescribed by your dietary program.

Right Food (a.k.a. right type of food): (1) Food that promotes good health and healthy weight. (2) Food prescribed by your dietary program.

Right Type of Food *(a.k.a. right food):* (1) A type of food that promotes good health and living in your healthy-weight range. (2) A type of food promoted or prescribed by your preferred dietary program.

Right Weight *(a.k.a. healthy weight):* Every weight that's in your healthy-weight range is regarded as being a right weight for you

Right-eating Communication *(a.k.a. right-eating-creating communication, right-eating-promoting communication, healthy-weight communication):* Communication that tells yourself — or your mind — to steer you toward right eating and healthy-weight living

Right-eating Day *(a.k.a. healthy-eating day):* A day in which your overall eating for the day amounts to right eating or non-overeating

Right-eating Focus *(a.k.a. healthy-eating focus):* (1) Time spent thinking about, talking about, pursuing, and/or enjoyably doing right eating and healthy-weight living. (2) Focus on right eating and healthy-weight living

Right-eating Mindset *(a.k.a. healthy-weight mindset):* A set of perspectives and feelings that steers a person toward achievement of right eating

Right-weight-promoting: Promoting living at one's right weight, or in one's healthy-weight range; used, for example, in the context of right-weight-promoting thoughts, feelings, decisions, actions, communications, foods

Self-reinforcement: The act of delivering reinforcement to oneself or to one's mind

Setback Reversal: The process of creating a progress action out of a misstep or a progress lapse

Startup Action: An action that's performed at the startup of a particular pursuit, and which installs into that pursuit a vital success driver

Stop-eating Signal *(a.k.a. don't-eat-it signal):* A signal from your subconscious mind that it's time to stop eating (for that eating session or meal). Most likely the most common, or #1, stop-eating signal is the full-stomach feeling.

Subby: (1) A nickname for the subconscious mind. (2) The nickname John Correll uses for his subconscious mind.

Subconscious Mind: (1) The part of the mind that is not the conscious mind. (2) The part of the mind that operates "behind the scene" or "in the background."

Succeeding Activity *(a.k.a. success activity):* An activity that contributes to creating a certain desired life-enhancing situation

Succeeding Day *(a.k.a. success day, winning day):* A day that contributes to creating a certain desired life-enhancing situation

Success : The act of creating a desired life-enhancing situation <u>and</u> deriving benefits, enjoyment, and fulfillment from it

Success Action *(a.k.a. winning action):* An action that contributes to creating a certain desired life-enhancing situation

Success Activity: An activity that contributes to creating a certain desired life-enhancing situation

Success Day *(a.k.a. winning day):* A day that contributes to creating a certain desired life-enhancing situation

Success Driver *(a.k.a. success factor, achievement driver):* A condition or activity that, when present, increases the likelihood of a person succeeding at a certain pursuit — or, more specifically, increases the likelihood of a person performing actions that contribute to creating a certain desired situation or outcome associated with the pursuit

Success Killer *(a.k.a. fail factor):* A condition that, when present, increases the likelihood of a person failing at a certain pursuit, or causes the person to experience needless hassle and difficulty in succeeding at the pursuit. Basically, any particular success killer is "the opposite" of a certain success driver.

Success Methodology (*a.k.a. achievement methodology*): An action plan that pertains to a certain pursuit and consists of specific actions that, when performed by a person, causes a maximal number of success drivers to be included in that pursuit, thereby resulting in easiest possible creation of the desired situation or outcome associated with the pursuit.

Success Process: An ongoing series of success actions aimed at creation of a common goal

Success Pursuit: A pursuit involving an ongoing series of success actions aimed at creating a certain desired life-enhancing situation or outcome

Success-creating Action: (See Success Action)

Success-creation Process: An ongoing series of actions all aimed at creating a certain desired life-enhancing situation

Success-creation: The process of creating success

Thank You, Keep It Up message: A special type of message delivered as a reinforcing response to someone who performed a desired action or created a desired result. This "someone" can be you (or your mind), another person, or God.

Under-eating: Consuming fewer calories than what your body is metabolizing, or "burning up," per day

Underweight Body Weight: A body weight that's below your healthy-weight range. An *overweight body weight* would be a weight that's above your healthy-weight range.

Undesired Weight Reading: (a) When in weight <u>reduction</u> pursuit, an undesired weight reading would be a scale reading that shows a weight <u>gain</u> over the prior day. (b) When in weight <u>maintenance</u> pursuit, an undesired weight reading would be a scale reading that's <u>outside</u> your healthy-weight range — typically a reading that's <u>above</u> your healthy-weight range.

Unguided Eating (*a.k.a. non-controlled eating, undirected eating, automatic eating*): Eating activity that's not guided by the eater, or eating that's done automatically and without conscious deliberation

Unhealthy Eating (*a.k.a. wrong eating, non-healthy eating*): Any eating that hinders good health or hinders living in your healthy-weight range — typically, overeating

Weight Control (*a.k.a. weight management*): (1) The act of creating an actual body weight that corresponds to one's desired body weight (a.k.a. healthy-weight goal). (2) The act of regulating one's amount of body fat for maintaining one's weight in a certain weight range

Weight Correction Day: A day in which you take immediate action to correct an undesired weight reading that occurred in a daily weighing. This action typically involves under-eating (total fasting or semi-fasting) for a 24 to 48 hour period.

Weight Failure (*a.k.a. non-healthy-weight living*): Living most or all of your days outside your healthy-weight range

Weight Freedom Method: (See Weight Success Method)

Weight Freedom: (See Weight Success)

Weight Maintenance: The act of maintaining one's body weight in one's desired weight range

Weight Management (*a.k.a. weight control*): (1) The act of creating an actual body weight that corresponds to one's desired body weight (a.k.a. healthy-weight goal). (2) The act of regulating one's amount of body fat for maintaining one's weight in a certain weight range

Weight Winner (*a.k.a. healthy-weight winner*): A person who's in process of creating weight success

Weight Success (*a.k.a. healthy-weight success*): Living most or all of one's days in one's desired healthy-weight range <u>and</u> deriving benefits, enjoyment, and fulfillment from it

Weight Success Action (a.k.a. weight winning action): An action that contributes to creating weight success. Examples of weight success actions include: the ten Startup Actions, the five Daily Actions, the actions described in the Weight Success Benefits Directive, and any of the actions prescribed in section B of this book.

Weight Success Actions Scorecard™: A scorecard for recording and scoring one's daily Weight Success Actions

Weight Success Benefits (a.k.a. healthy-weight benefits): The good things you derive from your weight success pursuit, or from living in your desired healthy-weight range

Weight Success Benefits Directive (a.k.a. healthy-weight benefits directive): (1) A directive that's delivered to your mind, and which describes certain weight success actions to be performed by your mind, including subconscious mind. (2) A directive delivered for the purpose of instructing your mind to perform certain weight success actions

Weight Success Day (a.k.a. weight winning day): A day that contributes to creating weight success

Weight Success Dynamic: A dynamic in which doing the Weight Success Method each day installs success drivers into one's weight success pursuit which, in turn, results in experiencing weight success (see also Lifelong Weight Success Dynamic)

Weight Success Empowerment: (1) Power or ability to create weight success. (2) The empowering of humans to create weight success.

Weight Success Methodology: An action plan that consists of specific weight success actions that, when performed by a person, causes a maximal number of success drivers to be included in a weight success pursuit, thereby resulting in easiest possible creation of weight success

Weight Success Method™ (a.k.a. healthy-weight method, weight freedom method): A particular success methodology for weight management, this methodology involving a certain set of ten startup actions and also a set of five daily actions consisting of weighing, reinforcement or correction, benefits directive, goal statement, and guided eating

Weight Success Mindset (a.k.a. healthy-weight mindset): A set of perspectives and feelings that steers a person toward achievement of weight success

Weight Success Pursuit: A pursuit involving an ongoing series of weight success actions

Weight Success Secret™: To succeed at lifelong healthy-weight living, do Weight Success Actions every day.

Weight Victor (a.k.a. weight winner): A person who succeeds at living most or all of their days in their desired healthy-weight range and derives benefits, enjoyment, and fulfillment from it

Weight Victory Action (a.k.a. weight success action): An action that contributes to creating weight success.

Weight Victory Day (a.k.a. weight success day): A day that contributes to creating weight success

Weight Victory Pursuit: A pursuit involving an ongoing series of weight victory actions

Weight Winning Action (a.k.a. weight success action): An action that contributes to creating weight success.

Weight Winning Day (a.k.a. weight success day): A day that contributes to creating weight success

Weight Winning Pursuit: A pursuit involving an ongoing series of weight winning actions

Weight-reduction Success Graph™: A graph for tracking daily success in weight reduction.

Weight-success-creating *(a.k.a. healthy-weight-promoting):* Creating or promoting achievement of weight success; used, for example, in the context of weight-success-creating thoughts, feelings, decisions, actions, communications, foods

Weight-success-creating action: (See Weight Success Action)

Whole-mind Dynamic of Healthy-weight Living: A dynamic involving applying one's whole mind (both conscious and subconscious) in the pursuit of healthy-weight living

Win-Day Calendar™: A calendar for keeping track of the healthy-weight success days, or weight success days, in each month.

Winning Action *(a.k.a. success action):* An action that contributes to creating a certain desired life-enhancing situation

World Weight Success Empowerment Series™: A collection of publications containing information that empowers people to achieve weight success

Wrong Amount of Food: (1) An amount of food that hinders living in your healthy-weight range. (2) An amount of food prohibited by your preferred dietary program.

Wrong Eating *(a.k.a. unhealthy eating, non-healthy eating):* (1) Eating that hinders good health or hinders living in your healthy-weight range — typically, overeating. (2) Eating prohibited by your dietary program.

Wrong Food *(a.k.a. wrong type of food):* (1) Food that hinders good health or hinders living in your healthy-weight range. (2) A food discouraged or prohibited by your preferred dietary program.

Wrong Type of Food *(a.k.a. wrong food):* (1) A type of food that hinders good health or hinders living in your healthy-weight range. (2) A type of food discouraged or prohibited by your preferred dietary program.

Yo-yo Dieting: (1) Ongoing alternating periods of dieting and non-dieting. (2) Ongoing alternating periods of weight loss and weight gain.

SECTION E:
INDEX OF SUBJECTS

Where to Go for What You're Seeking about Weight Success

F

Failproof reminder mechanism, 41
Failure cause awareness
    success driver #2, 24, 137
False assumptions that are sabotaging healthy-weight living, 146
False assumptions that are sabotaging weight success, 146
Fat gain
    primary cause of, 62
Fat-promoting factors, 20, 63, 146
    Big 5, 63
    list, 20, 146
    movement to discover, 20, 146
Feedback
    what it is and does, 26, 140
Feedback system
    most powerful one for healthy-weight living, 25, 138
    success driver #7, 25, 138
Feedback to the subconscious mind, 132
Feeling expressions and subconscious mind, 133
Flow, 162
    in the PERMA model, 162
Focus
    success driver #12, 26, 139
    what it is, 26, 139
Food, 39
    right amount, 39
    right enjoyment, 39
    right types, 39
Full-stomach feeling, 58

G

Getting input from God to fix a problem, 117
Goal reminders, 115
Goal-achieving knowledge
    success driver #9, 25, 138
Goal-achieving mindset
    success driver #3, 24, 137
Goal-achieving relationships
    success driver #18, 27, 141
    what they do, 27, 141
Guided eating, 56, 153
    and during-eating self-talk, 59
    ending over-snacking with procrastination tactic, 59
    how to remember 3-step process, 56, 58
    self-talk, 57
    step 1 – Communicate, 57
    step 2 – Believe, 57
    step 3 – Appreciate, 57
    three step process, 56
Guided eating process, 56
Guided-eating self-talk

    and acting as-if, 57
    and belief, 57
    and breaking the habit of overeating, 58
    and how to follow a stop-eating signal, 57
    how to do it, 57
    sample statements, 57
    two actions, 57

H

Habit of unguided eating, 64, 152
    easiest way to beat it, 155
    how it comes about, 64
    it vs. you (wrestling match analogy), 155
    solution to, 154
Habit-driven eating, 153
Habits, 153
    action-habit component, 153
    consist of two components, 153
    mind-habit component, 153
    what makes them strong, 153
Half-canoe analogy, 29, 142
Healthy-weight Goal Statement
    nighttime iterations, 110
    waking-up iterations, 110
Healthy-weight living
    and family and friends, 121
    and negative reaction of others, 121
    and schadenfreude, 121
    and using your whole mind, 28, 142
    as a role model, 169
    as an opportunity to help others, 169
    benefits beyond weight success benefits, 168
    biggest obstacle to, 146
    I Am Healthy-weight Living story, 172
    nationwide, 182
    roadblocks to, 146
    the key to, 129
    way to nationwide, 182
Healthy-weight range, 36
    ascertaining ideal weight, 76
    be wary of other's opinion, 78
    definition, 76
    determining the span of, 77
    diseases it helps avoid, 79
    full explanation of, 76
    guidelines for setting, 76
    how living in it helps others, 81
    how living in it is a role model, 81
    in Weight Success Benefits Directive, 85
    mandatory feature of existence, 36
    setting upper and lower limits, 77
    when to change, 78
    why it's a key to healthy-weight living, 76
High-frequency focus statement, 110

Y

Weight Success Benefits Directive

INSTRUCTIONS: Use this Directive for Daily Action 3. ● Where there's a dotted line (............), say the name you use when speaking of or to your subconscious mind. ● Read this directive aloud <u>and</u> say it with some emotional intensity. (Reading aloud is best, but when you can't do that, whisper it to yourself.) When reading it, **strongly desire** for the actions it describes to be realized. And, **hold the belief** and act as-if what's described in this statement is *in the process of happening.* After reading the list of weight success benefits, for at least 30 seconds **visualize** at least one of the benefits as an accomplished fact. As you go through the day, *continue* believing and acting as-if what's described in this directive is in the process of happening. ● For set-up, insert your healthy-weight range and preferred dietary program into the blanks. For the "pounds–kilos" phrase, draw a line through the word that doesn't apply. List your weight success benefits on the lines at the end. Hint: Use pencil, not pen. Or, type it up and tape it in. (For more, see the Detailed Instructions for Weight Success Benefits Directive chapter, page 85.)

*   *   *

..........................., I want you to do these five very important actions, today and *every* day for the rest of my life.

1 – Guide me to *easily* living in my **healthy-weight range,** which right now is

_____ to _____ pounds–kilos.

2 – Guide me to *fully* doing my **preferred dietary program**, which right now is the

_____ program.

3 – When I say my Healthy-weight Goal Statement while eating, automatically create thoughts and feelings that guide me to Right Eating, that guide me to eating the **types** of food and the **amount** of food that results in me living in my healthy-weight range.

4 – Whenever I make a decision to stop eating, make the urge to eat *immediately* begin to fade away for that eating session. And, if anytime I happen to accidentally overeat, create an uncomfortable bloated feeling that lasts for a short time.

5 – Whenever I say my Healthy-weight Goal Statement, bring to mind a thought of at least one of my weight success benefits. And, then, create within me a *happy, positive feeling.*

The Weight Success Benefits I gain from living in my healthy-weight range include:

1. A greater chance of *living healthier longer* — or greater chance of living free of debilitating accidents, illnesses, diseases, and bodily malfunction.

_____

_____

_____

_____

_____

_____

_____

_____

_____

_____

_____

_____

_____

_____

_____

_____

_____

_____

_____

_____

_____

_____

_____

_____

I thank you, God, for the opportunity to live my life this way.

......................., please do *everything you can* to assist me in creating lifelong healthy-weight living in a positive, pleasurable way. This benefits me *greatly*. I realize you're now doing it, and I thank you for it.

Living in my healthy-weight range is a *mandatory,* <u>must</u>-have feature of my existence. I am doing it *now* and for the rest of my life — and doing it *easily* <u>and</u> *enjoyably*. Yes! Yes! YES!

*   *   *

NOTE: After delivering the directive, close your eyes and say your Healthy-weight Goal Statement <u>three</u> times. Do it with intensity. ~ Plus, each day allow yourself to get a *good feeling* from making your weight losses stick and from having realized healthy-weight living. You deserve it. It's a substantial praiseworthy achievement.

> The **Weight Success Benefits Directive** is an important message for your mind, especially your subconscious mind. Deliver it like it is and your subconscious mind will act accordingly.